Splits Method

The Ultimate Beginner's Splits Stretching Flexibility Guide - Safe & Easy Splits Exercises Guide to Stretch Painlessly (No Machines, Cables or Equipment Needed)

By *Freddie Masterson*

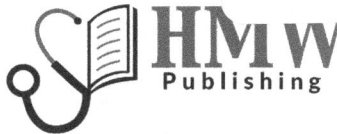

I0145777

HMW Publishing

For more great books visit:

HMWPublishing.com

Download another book for Free

I want to thank you for purchasing this book and offer you another book (just as long and valuable as this book), "Health & Fitness Mistakes You Don't Know You're Making", completely free.

Visit the link below to signup and receive it:

www.hmwpublishing.com/gift

In this book, I will break down the most common health & fitness mistakes, you are probably committing right now, and I will reveal how you can easily get in the best shape of your life!

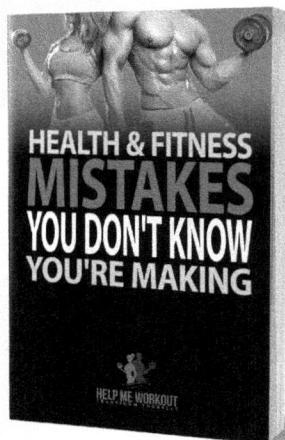

In addition to this valuable gift, you will also have an opportunity to get our new books for free, enter giveaways, and receive other valuable emails from me. Again, visit the link to sign up:

www.hmwpublishing.com/gift

Table Of Contents

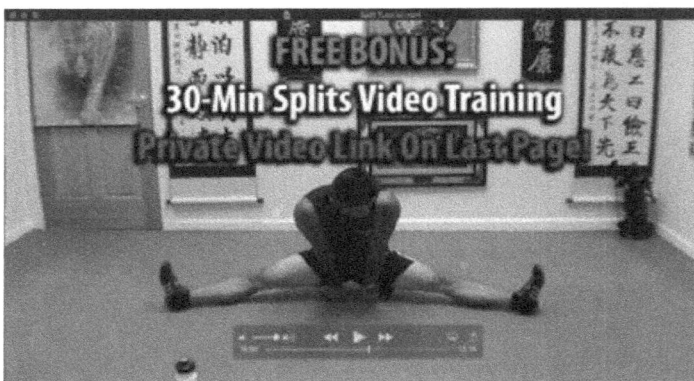

Introduction

I want to thank you and congratulate you for purchasing this book, "Splits Method". I'm glad to be able to share some ideas and secrets with you today that will help you achieve the dream of performing the perfect splits! Yes, this is something millions of eyes share in common. Let me tell you that the efforts by the majority have proven out to be a wild goose chase since most of the methods being practiced around the world today would burn your sweat, make you fatigued and grant you everything other than your dream of the "PERFECT SPLITS."

My methodology and the main purpose of this short but resourceful book is to make your body HEALTHY and FLEXIBLE in a dramatically uncomplicated and efficient way. I won't stretch this guide and bore you with all the literary talk and complicated discussions, so all the readers out there put a smile on your face because this book is concise yet it has everything that you need to know to convert yourself into becoming a perfectionist in performing the splits. So you must be asking yourself: "Even if this book is an ideal one, what can be the minimum time it will take me to achieve the splits?". The answer to that question is it really depends. It can take as little as a few days to a few months; it all really depends on your current flexibility level.

Moreover, my name is Freddie Masterson and I am the lead author of this book. Before writing this book, I have practiced this stretching technique for over the past TWENTY-FIVE YEARS. If you have tried to perform the splits for a while now and have been stretching regularly. This guide may even help you achieve it in as little time as a few days. You know your body more than anyone else and without any doubt, every person has a unique structure, so the time varies for every single person out there.

As far as what I have done my whole life, I consider this technique to be the BEST because, I have an in-depth experience of yoga, stretching exercises, stretching aiders. I've even bought leg-stretching machines worth 250$, so that I can attain the perfect splits. In a nutshell, I've tried every available option to accomplish the splits, but for me, nothing except this technique worked. I've achieved the best results using this method, and I have demonstrated this technique plenty of times in my martial arts classes.

Thanks again for purchasing this book, I hope you enjoy it.

Also, before you get started, I recommend you **joining our email newsletter** to receive updates on any upcoming new book releases or promotions. You can sign-up for free, and as a bonus, you will receive a free gift. Our "*Health & Fitness Mistakes You Don't Know You're Making*" book! This book has been written to demystify, expose the top do's and don'ts and to finally equip you with the information you need to get in the best shape of your life. Due to the overwhelming amount of mis-information and lies told by magazines and self-proclaimed "gurus", it's becoming harder and harder to get reliable information to get in shape. As opposed to having to go through dozens of biased, unreliable and un-trustworthy sources to get your health & fitness information. Everything you need to help you has been broken down in this book for you to easily follow and to immediately get results to achieve your desired fitness goals in the shortest amount of time.

Once again, to join our free email newsletter and to receive a free copy of this valuable book, please visit the link and signup now:

www.hmwpublishing.com/gift

Chapter 1 – Learning The Basics

It is important to learn the basics of SPLITS before we begin this undertaking.

Definition of the splits:

The split is the typical position of the body in which your legs are extended to their utmost but in opposed directions. Look at the picture below to visualize the side splits.

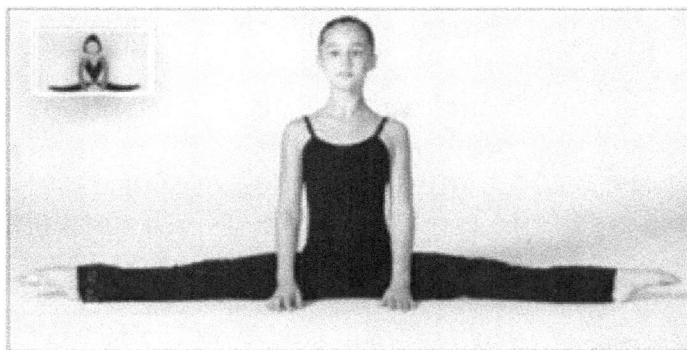

While performing the split the angle between the two legs is almost 180 degrees. Let's learn a little more about the basics of splits:

A split exercise involves the astonishing flexibility of three muscles: Iliacus – Psoas – Hamstrings

- **Iliacus** - As per Wikipedia - The iliacus is a flat, triangular muscle, which fills the iliac fossa on the interior side of the hipbone.

- **Psoas** - Psoas is a surface muscle, which most of us can't flex or release at will. It is s deep tissue involved in complex moves and interactions through the core and lower part of the body.

- **Hamstrings** - The Hamstrings muscles is comprised of three separate muscles, the Biceps, Femoris, and Semitendinosus. They are primarily fast-twitch muscles, responding to low reps and powerful movements.

A thorough knowledge of muscles is essential, but it is not mandatory to become an expert while we learn more about the splits. Splits can also be classified into a variety of types by the body orientation.

Here's a brief list of the different types of splits you can perform:

- Side Splits

- Over Splits

- Front Splits

- Vertical Splits

- Twisting Splits

- Half Splits

- Straddle Split Leap

Once you learn to do the side splits all the other kinds of splits come along very smoothly and without that much more effort. Side splits is the type of splits in which both legs are in the opposite direction concerning the trunk. You can scroll back to see the picture of Side Splits. We will now step into the core of the subject – "ISOMETRICS" – the prime requirement for achieving the splits.

Chapter 2 - Isometric Exercises

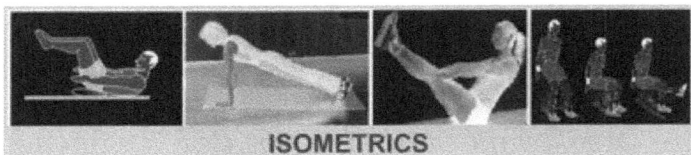

ISOMETRICS

We are slowly entering into the arena to perform actual side splits. If you have ever tried to do side splits, you should know the importance of muscle strength to perform it without pain. When your muscles are in firm position, you'll be putting a lot of command on your muscles. That command includes your WEIGHT and ISOMETRIC CONTRACTION.

Isometrics are a type of exercise training in which the Joint Angle and Muscle Length do not change during contraction. Isometrics is in contrast to concentric or eccentric contraction, which is typically called dynamic or isotonic movements. Isometrics is done in static positions, rather than being dynamic through a range of motion. Look at the figures above, and you will began to understand what are isometrics exercises.

Isometric contraction is a POWERFUL, EXTREME and MEANINGFUL contraction of the muscles that increase the length, force, and elasticity necessary for splits. You are doing this type of exercise style in order to FATIGUE your body rather than putting it in PAIN because fatigue is the main hindrance between you and perfect side-splits. Eventually, when you keep doing the isometric exercises, it will fatigue your muscles even more and leave them nothing but RELAXED, and this is what we want to accomplish.

My personal experience with isometric exercises

While I was in the Brazilian Jiu Jitsu demonstrations, our instructor made us undergo accurate control, weight and fatigue management. However, if our instructor caught us using our muscles or what I like to call "muscling methods." (Muscling is the utter dependence on muscle strength during grappling), he would have us go off to the side and do 50 push-ups. He would do this over and over again until our arms were so fatigued; we were incapable of "muscling" the techniques... even if we tried!

Muscling is NOT of prime importance because if you rely only on muscle strength the moment your muscles get fatigued you will surrender. Furthermore, by having our muscles so fatigued, we were forced to use leverage and proper technique!

What is proper technique?

This is what we call "isometrics." It protects our muscles against injury. The resistance of the three muscles is what makes the splits so difficult to attain. Striving hard to accomplish side splits but our hopes shattered, we start looking for MIRACLES.

We buy expensive stretching machines worth almost $250.00 and expect that agonizing ourselves will lead to any betterment in our progress with the side splits, which could cause permanent detriment to your muscles. I don't want to be sarcastic at all but this is what almost every one of us did including ME, and we failed poorly.

Isometrics on the other hand, repairs the muscles the same way as weight training. Isometrics makes the muscles stronger, more flexible, and ELONGATES them. We will proceed to SIDE SPLIS now. However, before we do that, it's necessary to summarize the key points of the above paragraphs.

- Isometric is a type of exercise training in which the joint angle and muscle length do not change during contraction.

- If you keep doing isometric exercises, it will fatigue your muscles even more and leave them nothing but RELAXED, and this is the primary requirement of achieving the side splits

Chapter 3 - Always Warm Up First

"To improve range of motion and avoid injury, you do need to stretch, but don't ever do it when muscles are cold." - William Levine, MD, Orthopedics surgeon and director of sports medicine at Columbia University Medical Center in New York City.

You must start your warm up with some light aerobic free hand exercises to get the blood to your muscle tissue and before doing any stretching.

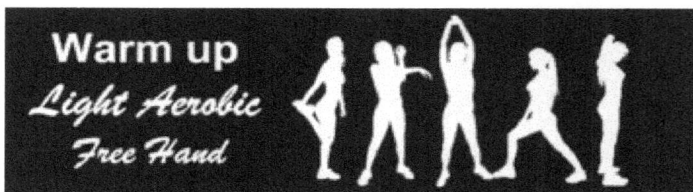

Why do you need to warm up?

Warm-up exercises are crucial before you do any workouts, or try to qualify for the above test - "Test your Potential." Preparing the muscles and joints for more intense activity will prevent injury, and promote blood circulation. Warm-up exercises increase the temperature of the body and make the muscles more flexible and receptive to strenuous activity. An overwhelming number of experts will agree that you should first do warm-up exercises before stretching. Warming up should increase your heart rate but not to the level experienced during actual SPLITS.

Do the usual exercises that you do to warm and loosen up your muscles. Start from simple jogging to stretching. WARM UP your body to let your muscles relax especially the hamstrings and iliopsoas. These can specifically be termed as the "Muscles of the back of the thigh."

It's important to know the limits of warm-up exercises.

You must listen to your body. If you are feeling tired, uncomfortable or notice a decrease in performance, you may need more recovery time or a break from warm-up altogether. If you are feeling active, you do not force yourself to do the exercises slowly.

If you pay attention, your body will let you know what it needs and when it needs to stop.

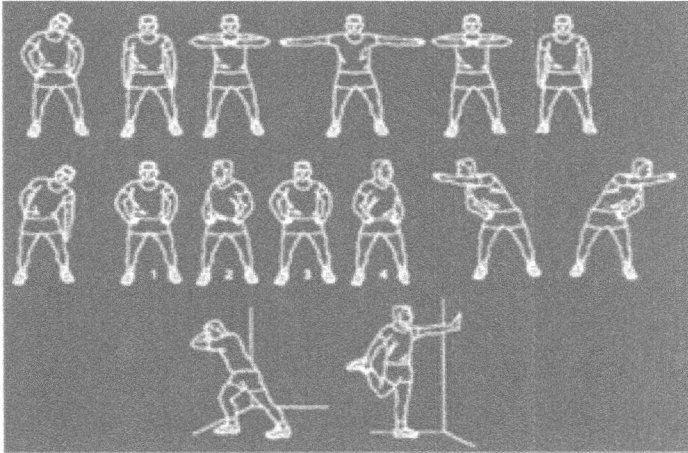

If you feel tired, it is better to do brisk walking or slow jogging for about ten to fifteen minutes, rather than stretching before exercise. The meaning of cooling down simply means slowing down, and never stopping altogether. Continuing to move around at a very low intensity for 5 to 10 minutes after a workout helps remove lactic acid from your muscles and may it will also contribute to reducing muscle stiffness.

What happens if you forget or don't stretch?

If by chance you forget to warm up your body, you will or could eventually damage your muscles, cause pain, and surely will not be able to do splits. Remember, the fatigue from the vigorous workout will allow your muscles to relax. A good warm-up prepares your body for more intense activity.

Warming up will allow your body time to adjust to the demands of exercise.

You should warm up for 5-10 minutes by doing some light exercises as outlined in the following chapter and **then** you should stretch. The reason for this is that stretching cold muscles can directly contribute to pulled and torn muscles.

Stretching, or should I say dynamic stretching will help your body to get ready for training. It's also an essential part of recovering from a warm-up activity. Again, you should switch to stretching after warm up and all training sessions should also end with stretching.

Chapter 4 - Test Your Potential

You must test your potential before you try to attempt a side splits. There are a few things that this book can't teach you, and testing your potential for the side splits is one of them. You need to do it yourself, as it is a self-evaluation process.

Your PELVIS is the only hurdle between you and you achieving the perfect side splits, unless you have some physical deformity. However, you should not worry, practice makes everyone perfect. Also, before you build up too much anxiety because of this test, let me relieve your tension. In my entire career, I have never seen anyone FAIL this test. We'll experiment the bony structure by performing HALF SIDE SPLITS.

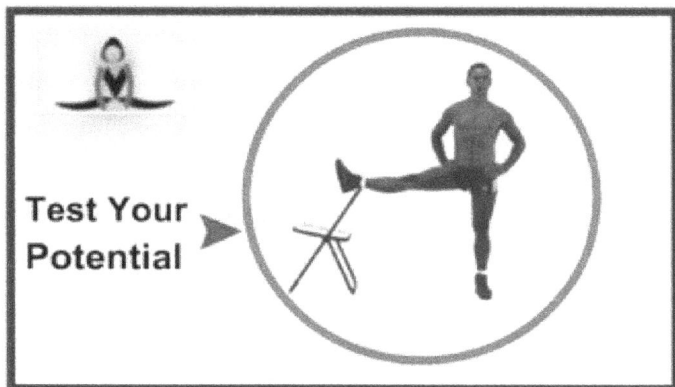

Test Your Potential

Step 1): Be sure to warm up and stretch your body.

Then position your body in such a way that your foot rests on a plane, such the height of plane equals your waist's height, e.g., on an Iron chair, a sofa, a table, a kitchen counter or some gadgets that suits you. It's also best to perform this in front of a mirror.

Step 2): Now that you have appropriately positioned your body.

It should look exactly as shown in the picture above. This is a half side splits because your leg is at the right angle concerning your pelvis and is positioned away from the body.

Step 3: Now look at the mirror.

Observe if your stance is erect and upright as if your feet are resting on the ground with an upright body. At this point, your hips MUST BE ALIGNED, if you don't acknowledge a "BONE TO BONE" sensation it means you do have the potential for side splits. It is this bone-to-bone sensation that hinders the body to stand in an erect posture.

What have you done?

Yes, you have done "Half Side Splits" with both your legs. This is proof that your hip joints have all the necessary mobility to perform a full side split. You have also proved that both leg muscles are long enough to perform a side splits.

Now you can perform a side splits with both legs stretched sideways simultaneously.

Nothing other than your nervous system will detract you to do a perfect side splits. It's important to teach your nervous system the perfect stretching methods. Once you do this, you will be able to do side splits anytime. I'm confident that very soon you will be the one smiling while doing the side splits! Going forward, please follow this systematic guide without any preconception, as this will help you gain momentum and allow you to progress faster.

Chapter 5 -Stretching Exercises

As we mentioned earlier, you should also switch to stretching after warm up. This will improve your ability to perform side splits. Once your muscles are warm, spend a few minutes on stretching. Since the goal of your warm-up is to increase your heart rate and get ready for a more intense job of side splits, you can choose a stretch that suits your body and workout environment.

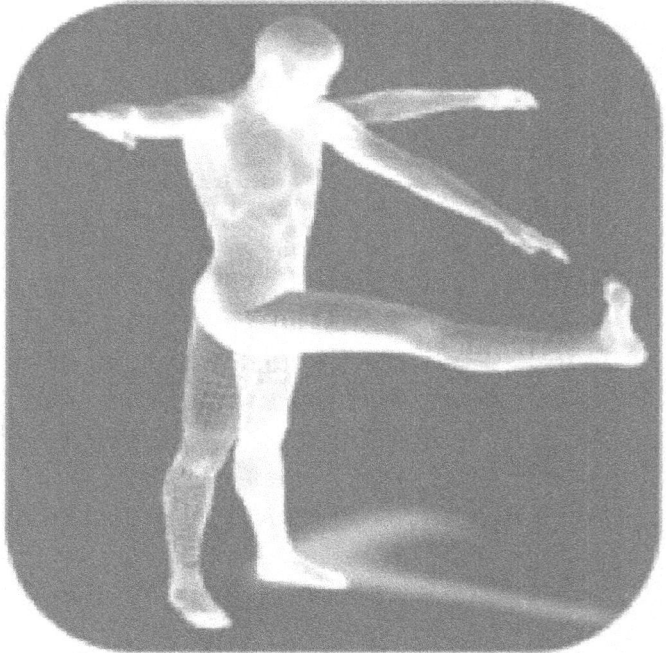

Dynamic Stretching

What is Dynamic Stretching?

Dynamic stretching means slow and controlled movements. It may include simple movements like arm circles, hip rotations, yoga-type movements, and some form of jogging or walking. The three pictures below highlights some postures of different stretches.

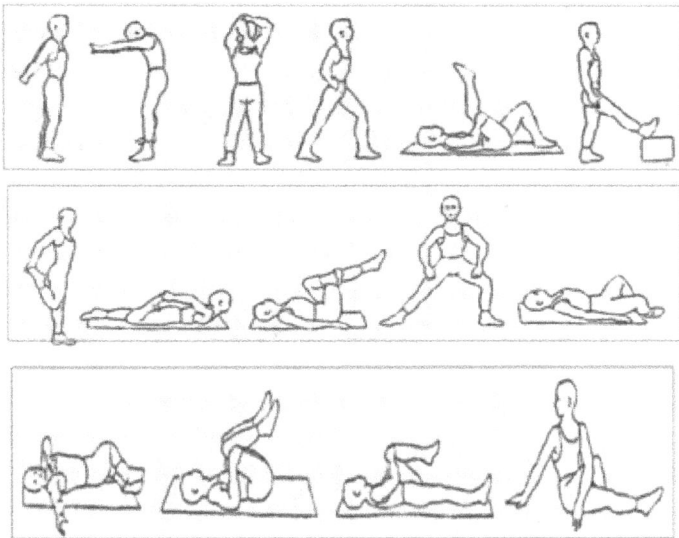

Here's some simple fixtures required for stretching exercises:

- Floor mat or carpet for comfortable sitting.

- Table or similar furniture to support your body weight initially.

- Shoes - wearing shoes is suitable for beginners.

- Stopwatch to measure your performance.

Stretching is the key element to help lengthen and loosen your muscles. Stretching is not the first thing you should do before exercising. I'm purposely repeating myself, however I cannot stress this enough. You should always warm up for 5-10 minutes by doing some light exercises and **then** you should stretch. The reason for this is that stretching cold muscles can directly contribute to pulled and torn muscles.

I'll show you the simple methods to perform some select Stretching Exercises relevant to Side Splits. However, before we do that, let me just highlight a few important points of stretching.

A few benefits of stretching:

- Reduces muscle soreness after warm up.

- Accelerates muscle tissue healing

- Improves balance and coordination

- Improves posture

- Promotes muscle relaxation

- Boosts your bodies energy levels

- Relieves back and joint pain

- Reduces the likelihood of back pain

- Promotes total body relaxation and a greater sense of well-being

- Maintains lifelong flexibility

Performing side splits is a challenging operation. This is highly useful for gymnasts, dancers, and for practically any sportspersons. It requires an enormous amount of flexibility in the hamstrings, groin, hip adductors and lower back. Whether you are already flexible or notyou will find greater flexibility and range of motion if you stretch your muscles before and after performing a side splits.

Lastly, right before you get started stretching, I want you to pay very close attention and I want you to thoroughly read the following in order to make sure you avoid any injuries.

Precautions during Stretching Exercise (Read carefully):

- Don't force a joint beyond its normal range of motion as this could potentially lead to instability of the joint.

- Be extra careful if you suffer from osteoporosis or are taking steroids as the risk of fractures is elevated.

- Avoid aggressive stretching of muscles that you have immobilized in a splint or cast. Connective tissues lose their strength some periods of immobilization.

- Stretching needs to progress gradually. In some cases it may take up to several weeks of a stretching program before you see significant results, so don't rush it.

- You should not be experiencing more than some transitory discomfort after a stretching session.

- Any pain that lasts for more than a few days may indicate the presence of inflammation. The famous saying "no pain, no gain" really does not apply here.

- Avoid stretching if you have swollen or edematous muscle tissues, as they are more susceptible to damage.

- Avoid over-stretching if you have any weak muscles.

- Make sure you always continue to breathe during a stretch. Holding your breath can affect your blood pressure.

Here's important Stretching Exercises relevant to perform Side Splits:

(1)   Downward Facing Frog:

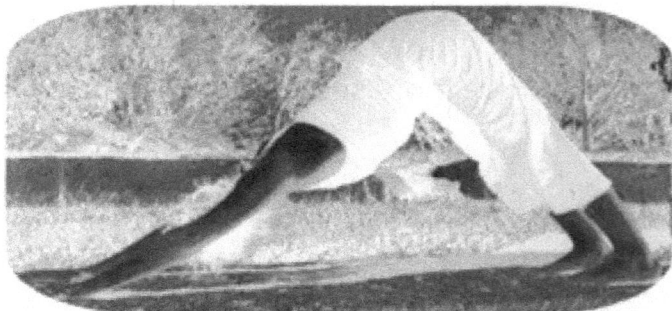

Downward Facing Frog

Downward Facing Frog is a deep stretching exercise for your groins, your hips, and your lower back. Position yourself on all hands and feet on the floor just like the picture, aligning your wrists under your shoulders and your knees under your hips. Open your knees as wide as possible and line up your ankles with your knees. Point your toes and feet turned out to the sides. Imagine that your legs are frog legs splayed out to either side. Rest on your forearms and drop your torso toward the floor. If you feel too much pressure on your knees, then put folded blankets or pillows before coming into the pose. Stay in the pose for at least 30 seconds to five minutes.

Instructions to perform this stretch:

(a) From Table position, tuck the toes under, press into the hands and begin to lift the hips up towards the ceiling.

(b) Spread the fingers wide apart with the middle finger facing forward, and the install your palms shoulder-width apart. Press the out through the fingers and edges of the hands.

(c) Using straight, however not locked arms, press the hips up and back reaching the chest towards the thighs. Lift yourself up through your tailbone to keep your spine straight and long.

(d) Have your feet are hip's width apart with the toes facing forward. Press your heels on into the floor feeling a stretch in your legs and on the back position of the legs. The legs should also be straight, or you can have a small bend in your knees to keep the back flat.

(e) Let the head and neck hang freely from the shoulders or look up at the belly button.

(f) Hold your breath and do this for at least 4-8 breaths.

(g) To release: bend the knees and lower the hips back to Table position, or come all the way down to child pose.

(2)   Seated Straddle Stretch:

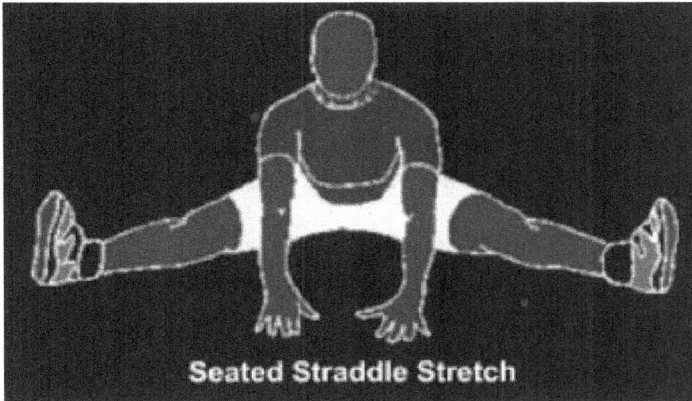

Seated Straddle Stretch

In Seated Straddle Stretch, you will stretch your groin, hamstrings and lower back muscles. Sit on the floor and make sure to keep your spine straight and your legs extended on the floor in front of you. Spread your legs and attempt to put them as wide as possible making a "V" shape, also make sure your knees and toes pointing towards the sky. Engage your core muscles by flexing your belly button inward your spine and lengthen through your spine. Hinge at the waist and fold forward, lower your torso and make sure it is toward the floor. Hold this stretch 30 seconds to 5 minutes.

(3)   Butterfly Stretch:

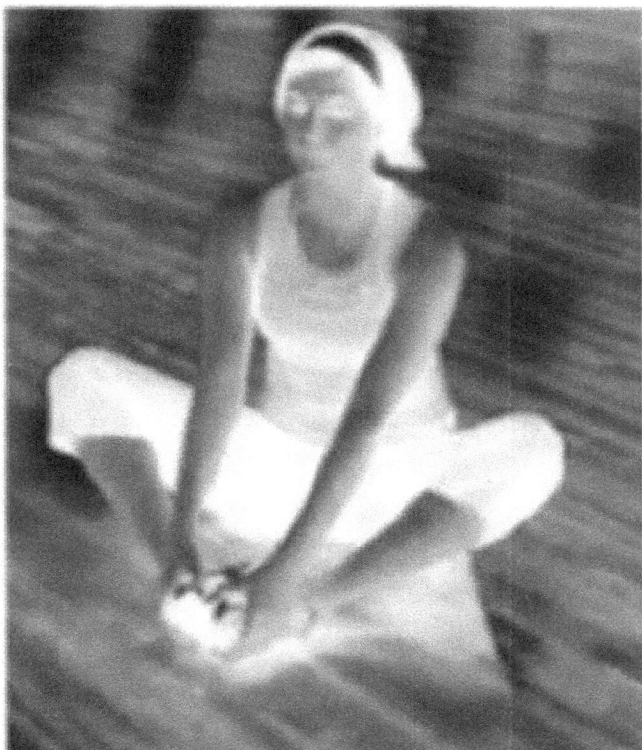

The Butterfly Stretch targets the inner groin, hips and lower back muscles. To perform this stretch, make sure you are sitting up tall with a straight spine. Also make sure to bend your knees, press the soles of your feet together directly in front of your groin. Hold on to your toes with both of your hands. Hinge forward towards your waist and lower your torso as much as possible down toward the floor.

Press the feet into each other firmly to encourage your hips to open up even further. Hold your stretch movement for 30 seconds up to 5 minutes.

(4) Hip Adductor Stretch:

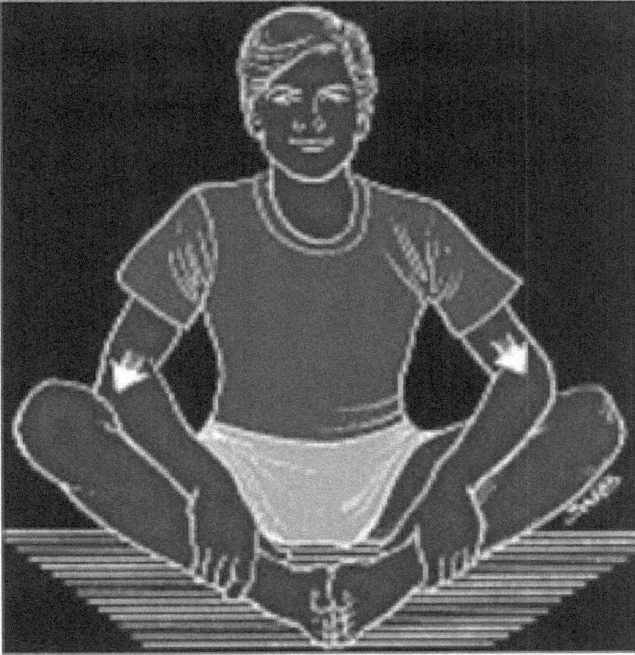

Sit on a firm surface and place the soles of

your feet together forming a circle with your

legs. Gently lean forward to feel your inner

thigh stretch. For a stronger stretch, use your

arms to push your knees gently toward the

floor. Hold your position for 15 to 30 seconds. This stretches the hamstring. Repeat this exercise at least 5 times.**Bent leg calf stretch**

(5) Bent leg calf stretch

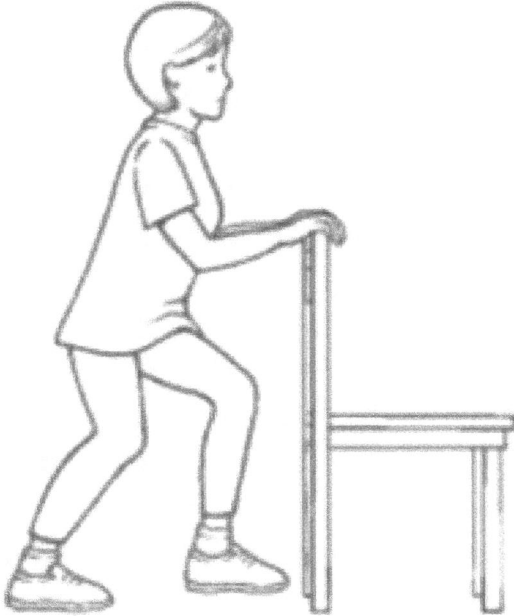

- Lean against a wall, tree, or chair for support.

- Place your right foot back; make sure to keep your toes pointing forward.

- Slightly bend your left knee, never letting it go beyond your toes.

- Slowly bend your right knee while you are doing this.

- Keep your head up and spine straight.

- Press your heel of the right foot to the ground.

- Hold and then repeat with the left leg.

(6)Front of calf and toe stretch:

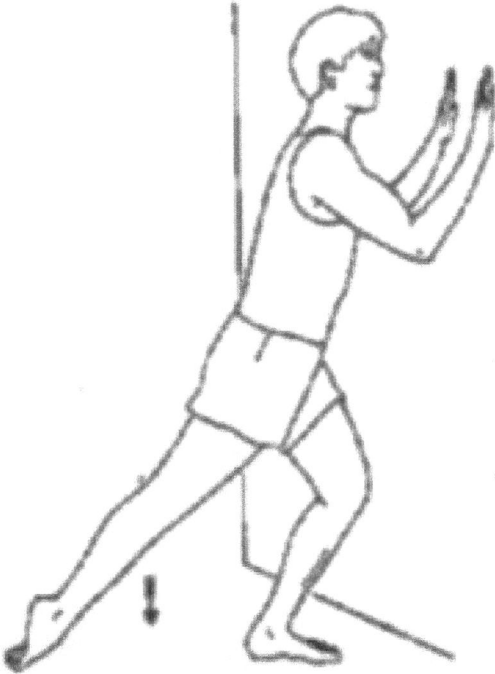

- Lean against a wall, tree, or chair for support.

- Bend your left knee and make sure never to let it go beyond your toes.

- Put your right leg back with your toes pointing straight backward.

- Keep your head up and spine straight.

- Gently press the front of the back foot and lower leg toward the floor.

- Hold and then repeat with your left leg

A great tip you should keep in mind while stretching

Stretch your body until it is fatigued. You should not put yourself in pain. If you feel pain, then your body is not sufficiently tired.

Extensive documents are covered in Chapter – 3- "Always warm up first" and here Chapter – 5 – "Stretching Exercises."

Read the chapters carefully, and master theses stretches. Try both the exercises. If you could not pass – Chapter - 4 –"Test your potential" try now, and I'm confident that you will pass the test.

Chapter 6 - Stretching:

Preparation to do Splits

Our mission is for me to teach you Splits through this book. You will notice that I have introduced representative images in every chapter. I believe you can do Splits with this guide, but you need to read it several times and practice the exercises by following the images, till you can perform your selected tasks at ease. We're very close to learning the technique of doing Splits. You have to master this chapter because you have to achieve easy stretching to learn the splits.

There are two types of splits, the Side Split, and Front Splits. Both these splits will demand considerable flexibility in your lower back, hamstrings and inner thighs. I've shown you a series of preparatory Stretching Exercises in "Chapter – 5- Stretching Exercises". Before you try to stretch yourself to learn to do the splits, you must attain the required flexibility through stretching exercises. This is the primary requirement for a fruitful and painless Split.

Reminder for "Preparation-Exercises" before Splits:

Warm up with a 10-minute exercise – see – Chapter -4 – "Always warm up first."

Do "Seated Straddle Stretch-

(see Chapter 5)

Stand with your feet shoulder-width apart and your   arms by your side.

Swing your right leg up and try to touch your thigh to your chest.

Keep the leg straight throughout the movement and swing your arms to help your balance.

Do 20 repetitions and then switch legs.

Final Check: Have you achieved considerable flexibility in the lower back, hamstrings and inner thighs? If not, follow this Golden-4-Step Freehand Exercise, and you'll be ready for Splits:

Golden-4-Step Freehand – Step - 1:

- Lie on your back on an exercise mat. Keep your left leg straight and bend your right leg. Lift your right leg and bring your thigh as close as you can toward your chest. Hold the position and count to 10. Cross your bent leg over your straight leg and try to touch your knee to the floor while keeping both shoulders on the floor.

- Hold and count to 10 again.

- Repeat the same sequence of movements with your left leg. Bend both legs, keep them together and lift them toward your chest. Keep your back on the floor.

- Hold and count 10.

- Lower both legs, so your thighs form 90-degrees with your body and your feet are off the floor. Keep your legs together and knees bent and swing them to your left. Try to touch knees to the floor. Hold for 10 seconds and swing to your right.

These exercises will improve the flexibility of your lower back.

Golden-4-Step Freehand – Step - 2:

- Sit on an exercise mat with your back straight.

- Bend both legs and place the soles of your feet together. Get your heels as close to your groin as possible. Grasp an ankle with each hand and rest your elbows on the inside of your thighs. Gently push down on your thighs with your elbows and try to touch your knees to the floor. Hold the position and Count 10. Relax and Repeat five times.

- On the fifth time, lean forward and try to get your chest as near the floor as possible.

- Hold the position for 10 seconds, relax and repeat four more times. This stretches your groin, inner thighs, and lower back.

Golden-4-Step Freehand – Step - 3:

- Sit on a bench or couch.

- Place one foot on the floor and stretch your other leg out on the bench in front of you. Bend the leg on the bench slightly, lean forward and grasp the balls of your foot. Gently pull the balls and toes of your foot toward you until you feel a stretch in your calf.

- Hold and count of 20. Now relax for 2 minutes.

- Next, pull the balls of your foot more firmly toward you and simultaneously try to straighten your leg by pushing against your hand with your calf muscle.

- Do not straighten your leg. Hold and count 20. Relax for 2 minutes. Next, stretch your hamstrings. Straighten your leg, place your hands close to your heel, lean forward and try to touch your chest to your thigh.

- Hold for 20 seconds.

- Change legs and repeat the sequence of movements.

Golden-4-Step Freehand – Final Step:

- Perform the seated stretch.

- Sit on the floor with both legs stretched out to the sides as wide as possible. Lean to the one hand, bend from the hips and try to touch your chest to your knees. Hold for 10 seconds then lean to your other side and repeat the movement.

- Next reach forward with both hands, bend from your hips and try to touch your chest to the floor. Hold and count 10.

  Repeat the sequence of movements. This stretches your inner thighs, hamstrings, and hips.

(Note: You may use a partner to help you do the seated stretch. Your partner sits in front of you with their legs spread out wide and leans forward to grip your wrists. He positions each heel on the inside of your feet and gently pushes your legs out wider while pulling you forward).

- Hold the stretch and count 10.

- Relax for 2 minutes and repeat.

- Now you should be ready to do Splits.

Chapter 7 - Simple Stretch For Side Splits

The splits is one of those moves that is easy for some people and much harder for others. Even if you have tight muscles, you will still be able to master it if you work hard and continually stretch.

In this chapter, I will show you simple stretch movements for side splits. It will be wise for a beginner to master the "Simple stretches" first before moving on to "Advanced Full Split Stretches" in the following chapter.

Here is another small caution for you:

Be sure to do each stretch on both sides – you will want a good splits on both your right leg and your left leg. Also, do not perform theses stretches until you feel that you are ready to do so. Practice all the stretches mentioned previously to be as flexible as you can and only then gradually begin the stretches mentioned in this chapter. We want to avoid any injuries at all costs! Please follow the Illustration below.

Steps for Simple Stretch for side splits:

Step 1): Starting position for a Side Split:

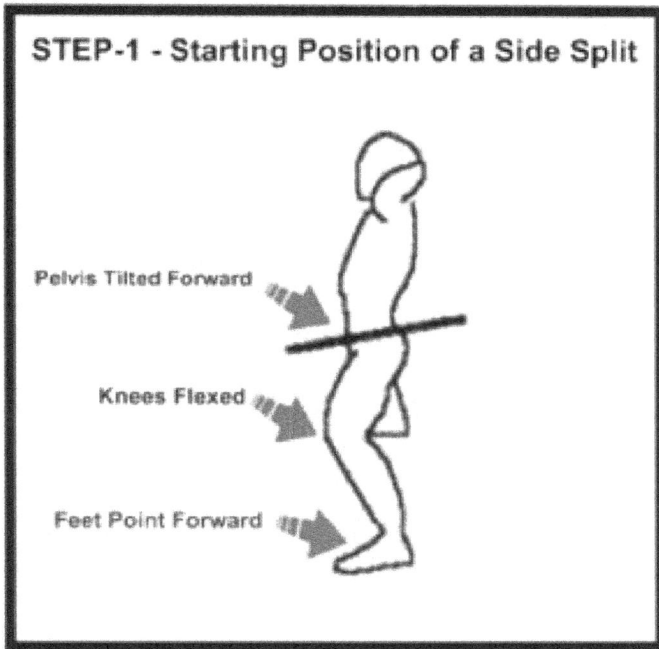

STEP-1 - Starting Position of a Side Split

Pelvis Tilted Forward

Knees Flexed

Feet Point Forward

- Make your feet to point forward

- Flex your knees as shown

- Point your feet forward as shown

- Repeat till you can do it at ease

Step 2): Beginning to get a Side Split

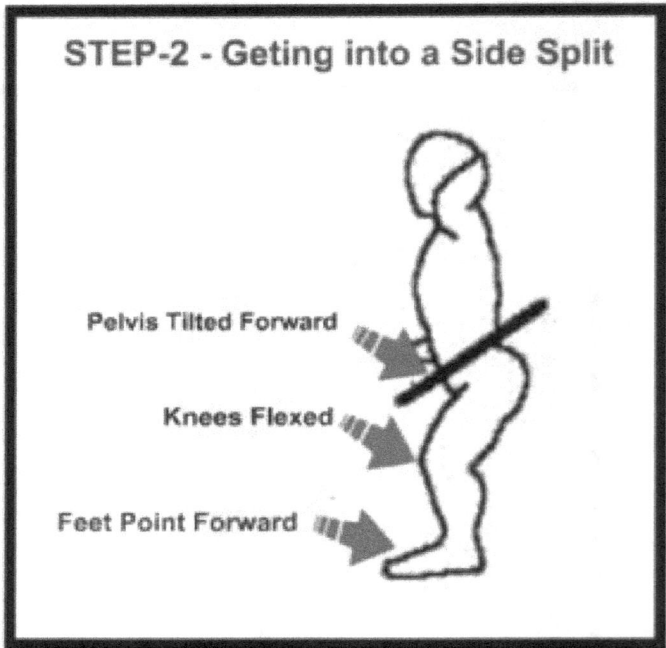

STEP-2 - Geting into a Side Split

Pelvis Tilted Forward

Knees Flexed

Feet Point Forward

- Spread your Legs sideways

- Tilt your Pelvis more as shown

- Point your feet forward as shown

- Repeat till you can do it at ease

Step – 3: Side Split with Feet pointing up:

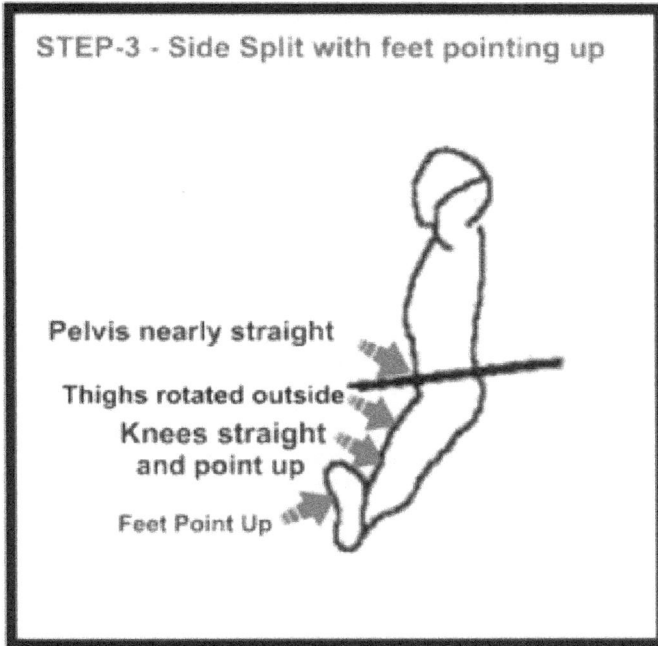

STEP-3 - Side Split with feet pointing up

Pelvis nearly straight

Thighs rotated outside

Knees straight and point up

Feet Point Up

- Make your hips straight

- Make your Pelvis nearly straight as shown

- Make your knees straight and pointing up

- Rotate your thigh outside as shown

- Repeat till you can do it at ease

Benchmark indicator

Now I've created a **Benchmark indicator** for you. Check your "Simple Stretch Side Split" performance after you have trained yourself in the above Three Steps.

(1) **See the figure below.** O.K! Keep your back upright and your pelvis tilted forward. Hips forward, and do not let you butt sag back on an upright side split stretch. If you can do this accurately, your Benchmark = 2.

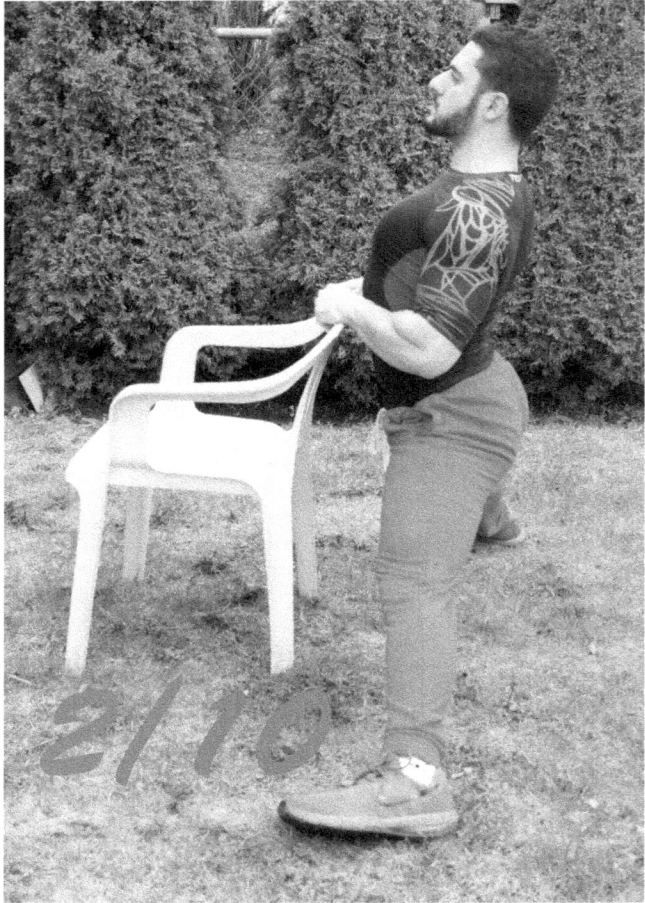

(2) **See the figure below** and make your ankles, knees, and hips in a straight line. If you can do this side split position correctly, then your Benchmark=4. Not a bad Benchmark.

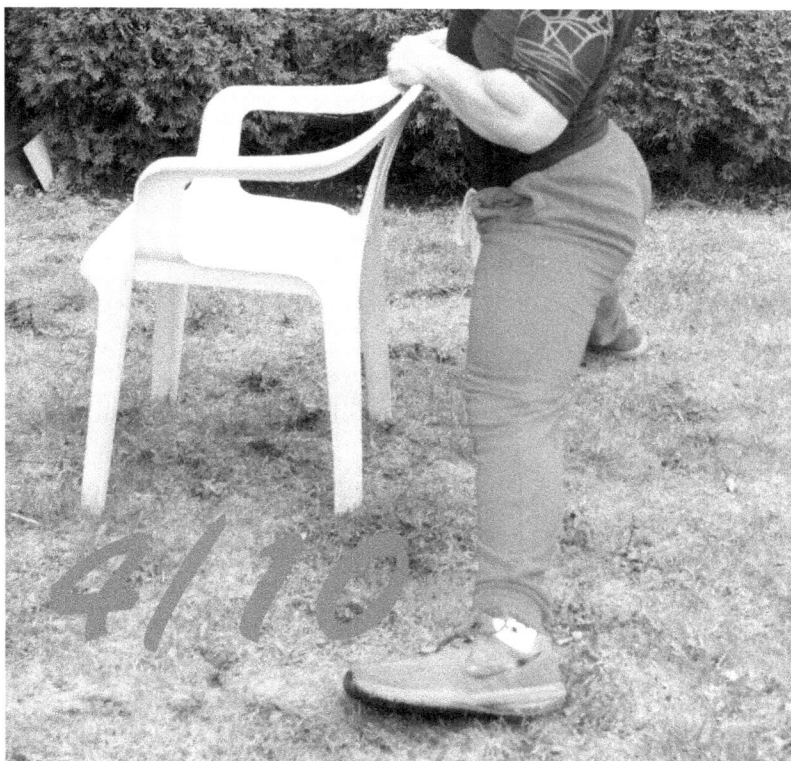

(3)   Look at the picture below, and maintain the position of your hips right up on the chair with the back upright and ankles, knees, and hips in a straight line. If you can do it easily and keep it for 5 minutes

after a few trials, your Benchmark=6.

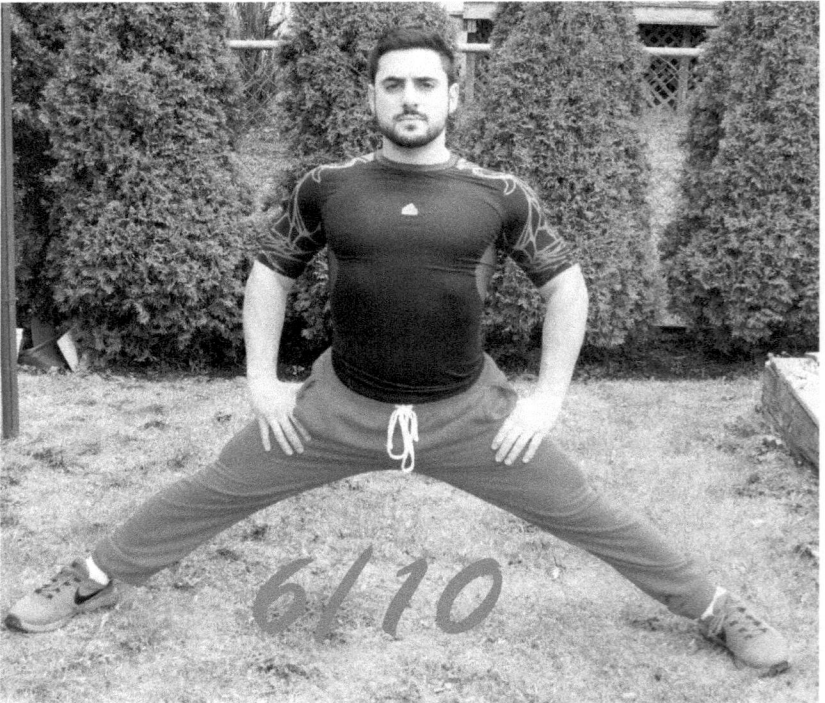

(4) **See the picture below.** You increase

your stretch and relax for at least 2 minutes.

If you can do it, your Benchmark=8. Keep it

up and proceed to get a perfect 10. Good Luck!

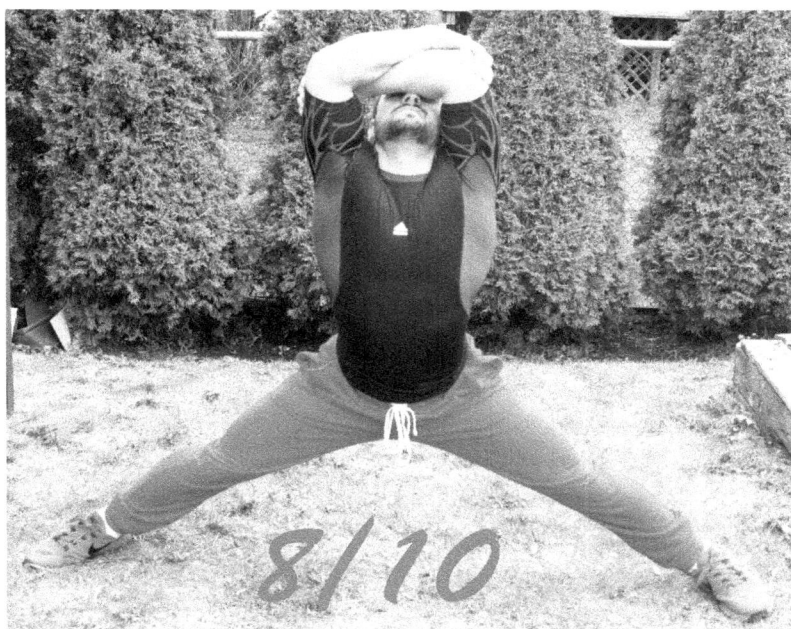

(5) Now, look at the picture below. This is the final position. If you can remain in this Side Split position for 5 minutes, your

Benchmark = 10 = Full Mark. Bravo, this is a

great success!

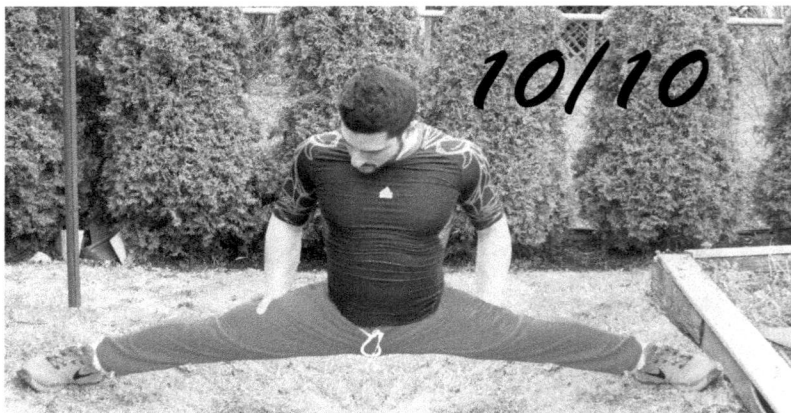

Chapter 8 - Advance Stretches For Full Splits

Once you have achieved 10/10 in the above Simple Stretch for Side Splits, you have to move to Advance Stretches for Full Splits.

Study the Illustration and try to imitate the postures below:

Posture – 1

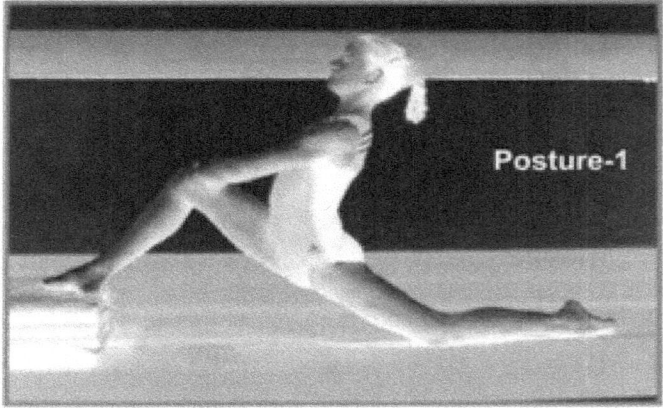

Posture-1

- To imitate the above Advance Stretch, a kneeling stance put one foot in front of you on a mat.

- On the other foot over a step, or some other object about **one foot** or more off the ground.

- Bend your leg to 90 degrees, and place your foot flat on the mat.

- Keeping your hips facing the mat, move the other leg facing backward, bending your knee behind you, until you form a "mini-split" from knee to knee.

- Push your hips forward as much as possible, working towards 180 degrees from knee to knee.

- Keep your chest up and your hands on your front knee.

- Attempt to hold this stretch position for about 30-60 seconds at a time. **Repeat this 3 to 4 times.**

Posture – 2

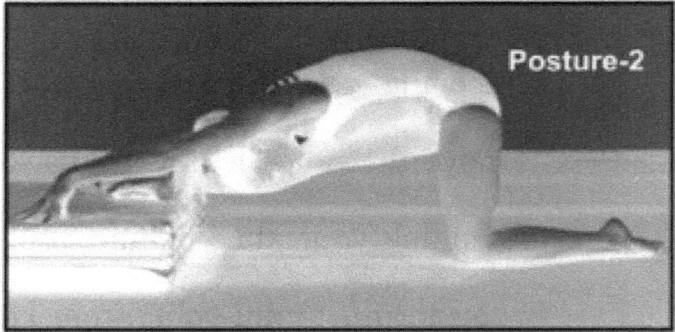

Posture-2

- Put one leg up straight in front of you onto the mat from a kneeling position.

- Move your body back, so only your heel is on the mat.

- Your back leg should be at a 90-degree angle, and your hips should be in a "square" position – they should

be facing the mat, not turned one way
or the other.

- Keep your front leg straight and lean
as forward as possible.

- Attempt to hold this stretch position
for 30-60 seconds at a time.

- Repeat 4 to 5 times till you can do it
easily and without any pain.

Posture – 3

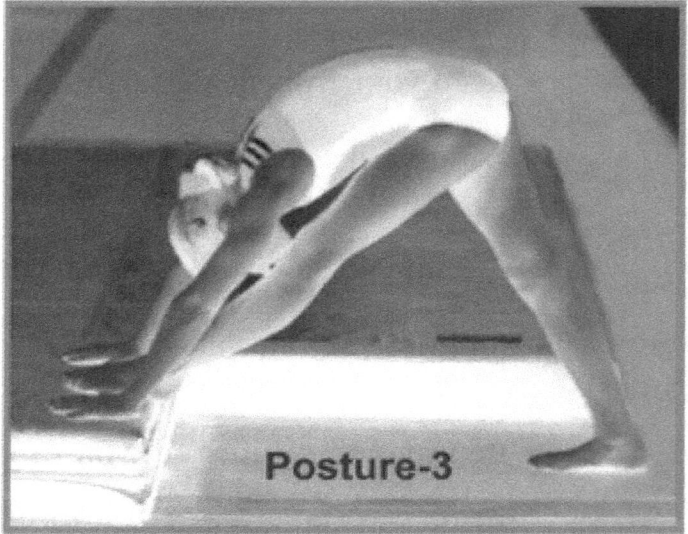

Posture-3

- From a standing position, put one leg on the mat in front of you.

- Keeping both legs straight and your hips square, lean forward as far as possible.

- Your back foot should be placed on the ground and your foot straight or turned slightly out.

- Repeat 4 to 5 times till you can do it easily.

Posture – 4

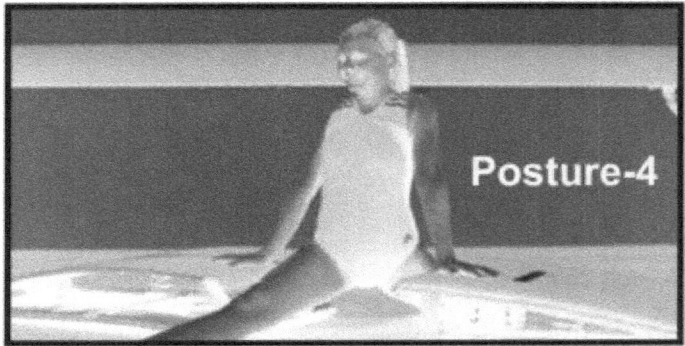

- You should keep your hips in a square position with your body.

- Your torso should be facing straight, and not to the side.

- You have to do it even if squaring your hips means you can't go down as far.

- Both of your legs should be straight and turned slightly outward.

- Your toes are to be kept in a pointed position.

- Your chest should be up, and not leaning forward.

- You can achieve this Posture – 4 with a little trial.

- Do it several times till you can perform this advance stretch quickly and easily.

Posture – 5

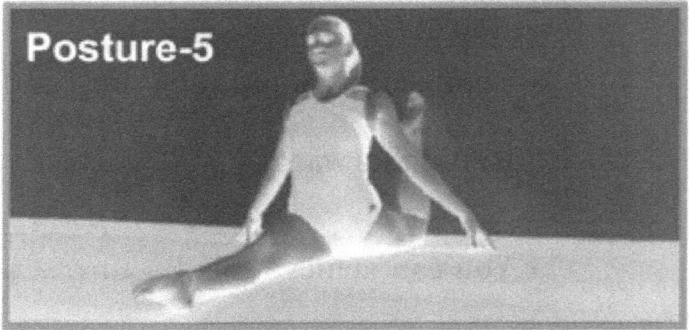

- In this Posture – 5, you have to make sure that your hips are square.

- It is best to try doing your split against a wall.

- Your back knee should be almost touching the wall, and your back leg should be bent at a 90-degree angle upward.

- Be sure that your back foot is pointing straight to the ceiling.

- You can also do this stretch with a friend holding your leg and helping you to keep your foot pointing straight up.

- Repeat this Split at least 4 to 5 times till you achieve perfection.

(Remember, you are very close to a perfect Splits).

Posture – 6

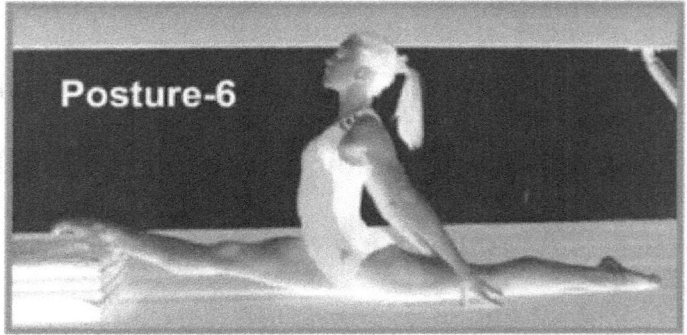

- You have already done a square split on the floor in Posture -5. See this position carefully.

- This is just a little advance pose, and just one step away from a perfect split. Now you have to put your foot on the mat. This will ensure your legs are over split or in other words a split more than 180 degrees.

- For even more of a stretch, do your split between two mats or two springboards.

- Repeat this split till your posture is just a mirror image of Posture-6.

Posture – Perfect

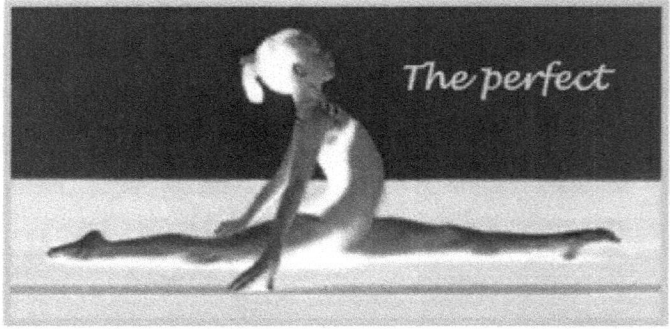

The perfect

This is "THE PERFECT SPLITS!"

Chapter 9 - Tips for 180 - Degree "Side Splits".

We have covered enough illustrative documents by which you can develop the required flexibility for a successful 180 degrees side splits session. However, you must read the documents, refer to Chapter 1 to 8, understand these techniques and try to develop your flexibility to meet the challenges of a Side Splits.

Side Splits requires less flexibility. I can assure you from my years of experience that if you stretch every day, you will likely see a lot of improvement in your flexibility. The Side Split is typically done facing forward with the legs extended out of the side in a 180 Deg. Split.

The Ultimate "7 Steps DAILY Stretching Exercises" to realize your goal of 180 Degree Side Splits

- **Step 1) Jog for 5 Minutes** to warm up your muscles – follow "Chapter -3 – Always warm up first".

- **Step 2) Stand on your feet shoulder-width apart** by pointing your toes slightly out. Bend your right knee. Slide your left leg out until you feel a stretch. Place your hands on the floor in front of you and maintain balance. Hold for 20 seconds. Repeat the same thing on your right leg.

- **Step 3) Stand on your feet with legs together.** Lower your upper body towards your leg – keep your legs straight. Wrap your arms around the back of your legs. Hold this position for 20 seconds. Reach your toes with your hands and hold for 20 seconds. This will stretch your hamstrings.

- **Step 4) Place your feet in a wide "V" Posture.** Lower down your upper body towards the floor, and remain there for at least 20 seconds. Now reach both hands to your left foot and attempt to hold it for about 20 seconds. Similarly, reach both hands to your right foot and hold for 20 seconds.

- **Step 5) Place your feet in a wide "V" Posture.** Twist your torso to the right and then bend your right knee to a 90-degree angle. Keep your left leg straight. Hold the position for about 20 seconds. Repeat on the other side to stretch the hip flexors.

- **Step 6) Sit on the floor with your knees bent** and the bottoms of your feet together. Lean slightly forward with a flat back. Pull your feet towards you until you feel the stretch. Hold for 30 seconds to stretch the gluteal muscles.

- **Step 7) Sit close to a wall.** Bend your knees and then place them on a mat. Slide your knees apart, so your thighs are in a "V" position. Your shins should be flat on the mat. Lean forward and place your forearms flat on the floor. Push your torso back toward the wall behind you. Keep your back flat. Hold for 20 seconds.

Chapter 10 - Contract & Relax

You have gone through a vigorous stretching exercise to achieve a 180 degree or 160 degree Side Splits. Now is the time to relax.

What happens when you stretch?

When you stretch, your nervous system activates the myotatic reflex or muscle contraction in response to stretching within the muscle. This is a stretch reflex – a mechanism of your body's natural defence against muscle tears. Your muscles will react when it feels they have gone too far. The good news is that you can train your reflex to fire much later, thus improving your pre-tensile range of motion, which determines how far you can stretch before your muscles tense up.

Contract and Relax training (CR Training) is an action in which all your muscles will go completely slack and remove all tension to avoid further injury.

Just follow these steps:

- **Step 1) Start your CR Training with the Horse Stance Position.**

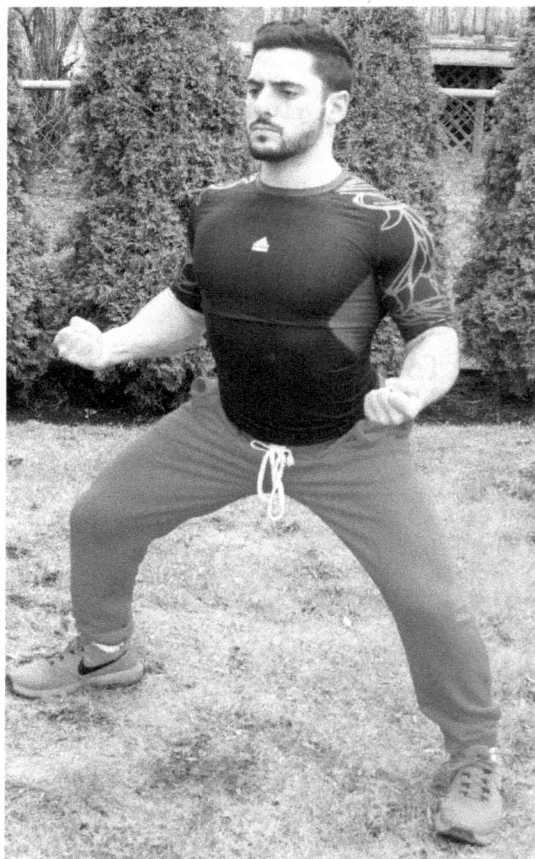

One easy way to assume this position is to stand straight up and bend your legs slightly. Place your body in such a way that your hands rest on your waist or hips, and your feet parallel to one another with straight back and knees bent. Now slightly start moving your feet far and farther away from one another such that it puts a stretch on the muscles of the back of your thigh.

If you are not at ease at this position for the first time, use some support to balance your body but remember the support is not to be used to bear your body weight. Keep your knees bent at all times during this "Horse Stance Position," because it is necessary to stress and fatigue your muscles and not your joints. The idea is to lock your knees and thus to sprain the knee-joint. You should feel relaxed.

• **Step 2) Gradually increase the stress on your muscles.**

You can do this by stretching them wide apart in HORSE STANCE POSITION. You will start feeling moderate tension. Remember, we are training your muscles to become habitual of stress and tension. You should not push yourself too hard to feel pain. Do it at ease and take your time. Be patient. You will feel relaxed by practice and over time.

- **Step 3) When you feel the first slight of stress, do this!**

Maintain your position when you feel the first slight of stress. Do not worry if at this point you have only wiggled your feet about a few inches, this is the first stretch, so this is the maximum you can do. While maintaining this position vigorously contract your muscles, enough that your legs start trembling. It happens because you are trying to move your legs close to one another and yet contracting them. Your legs at this point will look like two sharp ends of scissors.

HOLD YOUR CONTRACTION FOR AT LEAST 30 SECS AND TIME IT USING A STOPWATCH. DO NOT TOUCH THE FLOOR OR USE A SUPPORT TO BEAR YOUR WEIGHT. FOCUS THE WEIGHT ON YOUR LEGS.

OBSERVE: *At this point, your hands SHOULD NOT be on your knees, knees should be BENT and hips ROLLED. The level of ease of the next stretch depends on the duration of the first intense contraction.*

- **Step 4) Deeper Stretches**

After the first intense contraction maintain the posture for another 30 seconds and let your muscles relax. Perform a deeper stretch by moving your legs further apart to keep tension on your muscles.

This is the second contraction. Now after the second stress, STOP & CONTRACT AGAIN for another 30 seconds. When this contraction is over, RELAX your muscles and go for one more profound and intense STRETCH.

Now the third time when you are doing a stretch, and you can feel a CONTRACTION, hold this position for the same time span. This is the 3rd contraction. When this contraction is over bring the legs close to one another, shake them around, walk around and relax for 3-4 minutes. You will feel much better. Are you a bit confused?

• Let us **summarize the 4 Steps**:

THREE INTENSE CONTRACTIONS EACH HAVING DURATION OF 30 SECONDS MAKES ONE COMPLETE SET OF CONTRACTIONS.

• Align your body in horse stance position, move your feet apart causing your muscles to feel tension, STOP and CONTRACT for 30 seconds.

- Hold this contraction.

- Repeat this process twice till the third contraction is approached creating a DEEPER STRETCH.

- Stop pulling and RELAX.

RECOVERY TIME:

3-4 minutes, but don't stress your body this time can surely vary from person to person. So if you need more time to loosen up your muscles or relax, take that time because we don't want you to be uninspired by your progress.

- **Step 5) Complete a stretching session.**

  You can accomplish this by performing THREE TO FIVE TOTAL SETS OF CONTRACTIONS.

- **Step 6) Last Intense Contraction.**

  This Step is a modification of the last contraction and a little hard to achieve. This will also consume more time.

  Hold the very **LAST INTENSE CONTRACTION** for an exceptionally long time-span that is from **60-90** seconds. It is because of this duration that the last step is necessary for TREMENDOUS FINAL RESULTS because it is a strenuous task to accumulate the contraction for such an extended period of time.

Now carefully walk out of this stance and relax and loosen your muscles.

As you find yourself progressing with the stretching techniques rather than just dropping the method totally and giving it a fresh start every time, you should instead go with MINI CONTRACTIONS midway through the stretches.

1. Walk your feet apart until you have reached a few inches

2. Stop

3. Perform mini contractions for 3-5 seconds

4. Again walk your feet apart until you have reached a few more inches

5. Stop again

6. Perform mini contractions AGAIN for 3-5 seconds

7. REPEAT this whole process one more time

8. Keep doing it until you start feeling STRESS on your thighs

9. After feeling the pressure, do the EXTREME 30 seconds CONTRACTION.

Yes, you are done! You have successfully ELONGATED your muscles by REPEATED ISOMETRIC CONTRACTIONS.

Know the following truth about Relaxed Stretches:

- You can do Relaxed Stretches anytime, anywhere, and without any warm up.

- You must be patient while doing Relax Stretches.

- Never bounce in any stretch.

- Do Relax Stretches at the very end of the workouts.

- The optional frequency for Relax Stretches is once every day.

- Rotate your pelvis to prevent pain occurring at the top of your pelvis.

- Unlike dynamic stretching, it does not cause fatigue, which means even after an intense workout you can still, do a thorough stretching routine.

- It can be done any time of the day with or without a warm-up.

- It can be done by anyone regardless of his or her fitness level.

- It is the most enjoyable form of stretching and can leave you feeling completely relaxed.

At this point try to have 5 minutes for yourself to think about your expectations and how it is changing you now and in the future. We will now add some important documents relevant to "SPLITS METHOD."

Well, I feel that it is necessary to answer some relevant questions often asked by participants.

Chapter 11 - Practice Splits Every Day

When you do the splits, you spread your legs at right angles to your torso. As I mentioned several times before, to do the splits, you have to be quite flexible.

Your feet work best when your legs are spread against a flat surface. While some people are naturally more flexible than others, you can improve your flexibility with regular practice.

Practice the splits daily to see improvement

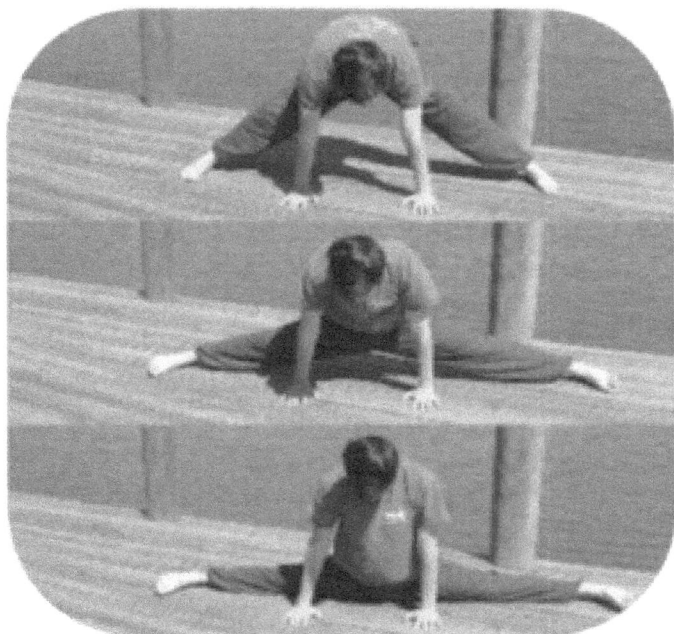

If you are still not able to do a full splits, practice stretching daily, and you will find you can spread your legs a bit farther each day – eventually to successful full splits.

- **Step 1):** Warm up your muscles by walking, jogging or performing exercises as outlined in Chapter - 4 – "Always warm up first" – Page – 15, or you may resort to some other cardiovascular exercise. If you do not properly warm up before attempting the splits, you may hurt yourself.

- **Step 2):** Choose which leg will be in front. Most people have more flexibility on one side. Find out your flexibility by trial.

- **Step 3):** Place one foot forward and the other behind you.

- **Step 4):** Slide your to away. You will slowly inch down toward the floor.

- **Step 5):** Use your arms to stabilize your body, as you get closer to the floor. Your hands should be placed on the floor for support.

- **Step 6):** Stop sliding when you feel discomfort in your legs. Do not continue if you feel pain. If you do, you may pull a muscle.

- **Step 7):** Remain in the splits position for a few minutes. This will help your muscles to become accustomed to the pose.

- **Step 8):** Practice the splits every day. You'll find you can get closer to full splits every time you practice.

You must record your daily progress, and hopefully, you will do the full sooner than you think! :)

Chapter 12 - Leg Stretches

I've purposely made sure to devote an entire Chapter on Leg Stretches. You may ask — why? Leg stretches are a critical factor of Side Splits, lower back health, and comfort. When the muscles of the legs become tight and short (it often happens due to sitting for long periods of time), they can fix the position of the pelvis preventing casual movement. When the pelvis is in a fixed position, the lower back can become strained, as it tries to compensate for movement.

What should be your goal be while performing Leg Stretches?

Your goal should be to lengthen the adductor muscles so that they do not prevent the natural movement of your pelvis during splits. Look at the pictures below.

Basic Leg Stretches Exercise

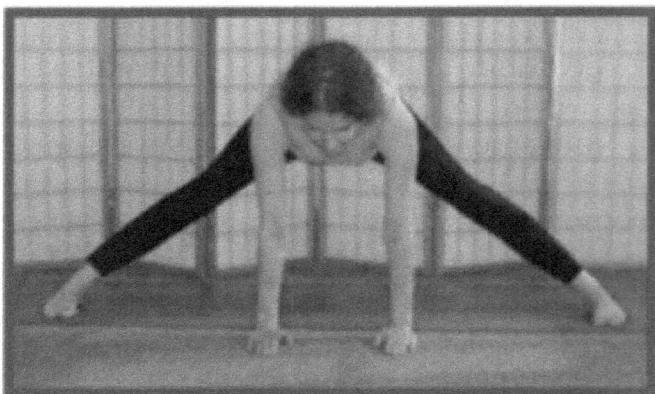

Gently ease down into a side splits. It's not important how far you're able to go. What's important is that you feel a comfortable stretch. Again, if you push your muscles too hard, they will rebel.

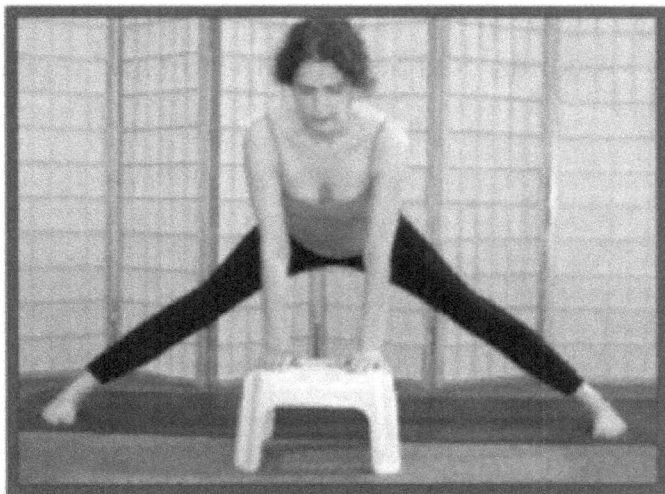

If you are not able to get your hands on the floor, use something else for support. See the picture on the next page.

If the above piece is not high enough for you, you may use a chair or even a countertop. Make yourself comfortable in this position, and then gently rock back and forth so that you will feel a rhythmic increase or decrease of the leg stretch. Don't spend longer than 30 seconds. It is best to come out and repeat it.

Leg Stretches for the Hamstrings:

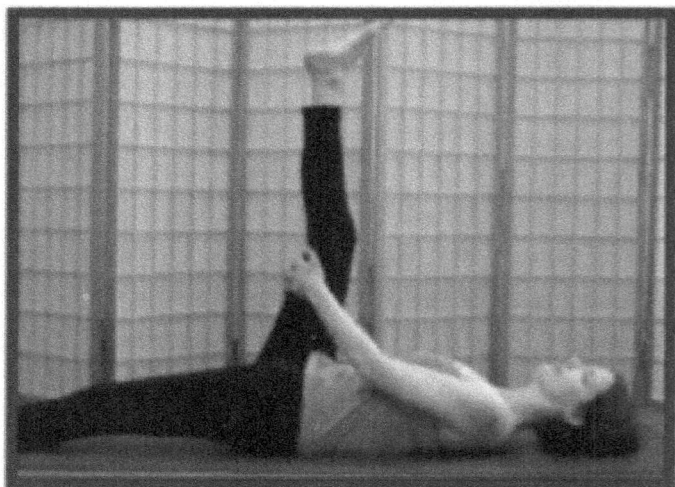

To ensure the comfort of the lower back and to prevent the progression of sciatica symptoms the hamstrings must undergo a regular stretch session.

Those who occupy a sitting position for much of the day are particularly prone to tight, short hamstrings. Tight hamstrings, like tight adductors, can exert a powerful immobilizing effect on the pelvis, which puts a strain on the lower back.

Lie on your back with one leg straight out on the floor. Grasp the back of the thigh of the other leg and straighten toward the ceiling. Don't worry if your leg doesn't straighten all the way! What's important is that you straighten as far as you're able to without too much strain, hold for just 2 seconds, then release allowing the knee to bend completely. Now repeat 10 times.

Two things likely distinguish this stretch from hamstring stretches you've done in the past:

1. You're not trying to stretch the hamstrings while holding up your body weight such as you would in a standing position

2. You're not holding the stretch for longer than 2 seconds. Instead, you're repeating the stretch 10 times.

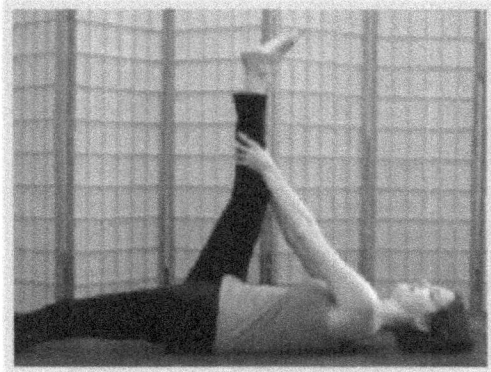

For very tight hamstrings I have found that this strategy is far more effective than static stretching in which the stretch is held for, say, 30 seconds. For those who wish to get a deeper stretch reach up higher on the leg during the lengthening phase as shown in the picture here.

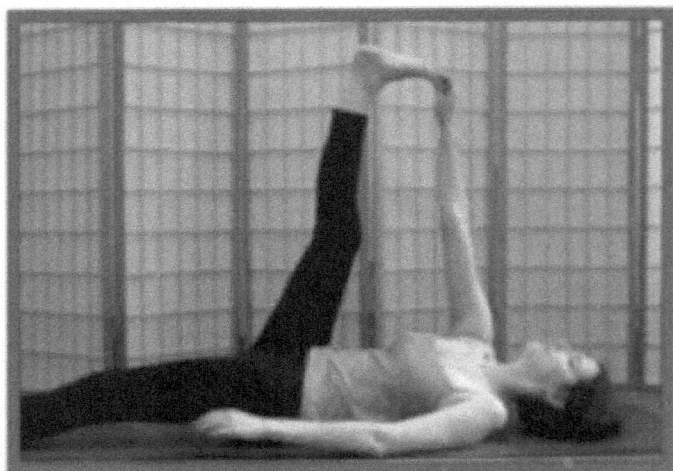

See the picture above. You can reach for the deepest stretch for the foot during lengthening process as shown in the picture here.

Leg Stretches for the Quadriceps:

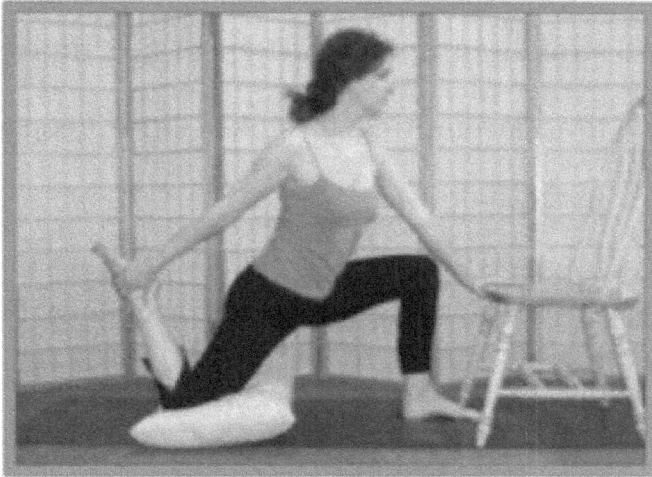

My goal is to lengthen the quadriceps muscles (the front of the upper thigh) so that they do not pull the pelvis into an anterior torque, which can strain the lower back.

The Kneeling Version: Begin in the supported position as shown in the picture above. Now bend forward while retaining a hold on the ankle so that you feel a deepening of the stretch into the quadriceps. Hold no longer that 1-2 seconds then straighten up again. Repeat 4-6 times, each time attempting to sink a little deeper into the stretch.

Switch legs and repeat this sequence. See the picture below:

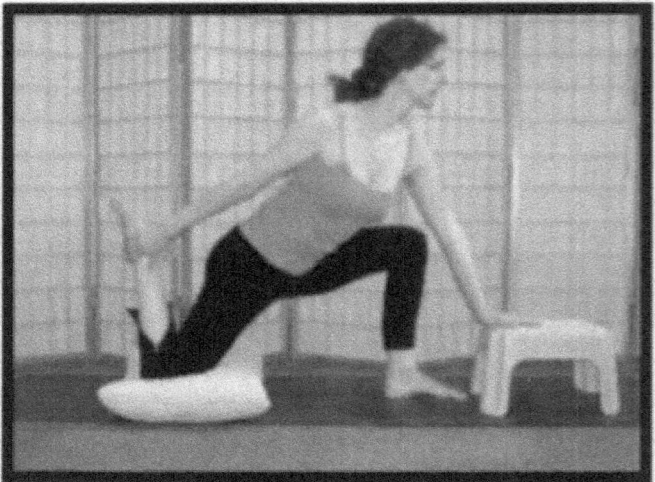

The Side-lying Version:

Begin in the side-lying position shown in the next page the image.

Now reach back with the left knee while stabilizing the left ankle and hold for no longer than **1-2 seconds** (Do not try to hold longer as it develops fatigue).

Repeat reaching back, feeling the quadriceps stretch for just 1-2 seconds, and then returning to the starting position. Repeat 4-6 times.

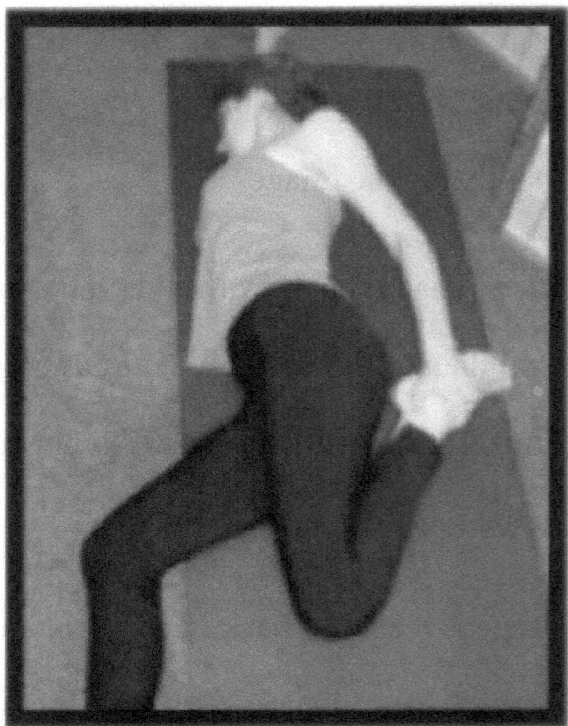

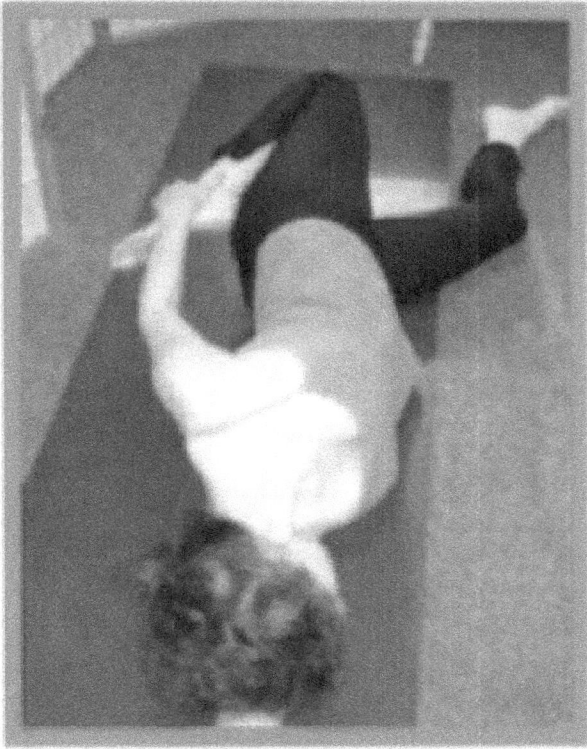

Repeat entire sequence on the other side as shown in the picture.

How to Improve Your Flexibility Safety During Splits.

Again, I cannot repeat this enough times. You should not make the common mistake of trying to push too hard during stretches. While doing so, you will risk tearing your muscle fibers. Muscles have a protective response called "Stretch Reflex" which makes the muscle contract during hard stretches. Thus pushing too hard has a detrimental effect. You will not get the desired result and at the same time risk tearing your muscles. So, the best technique is to do stretches gently and gradually over an extended period of time.

Bonus Chapter: Video

Stretching Tutorial

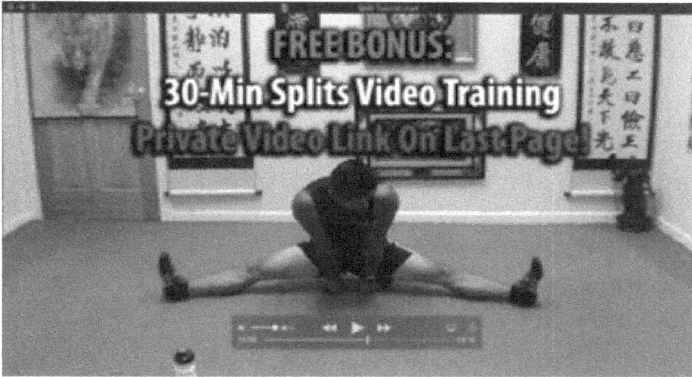

http://

www.hmwpublishing.com/

splitsbonus

Please DO NOT share this video. This is an unlisted video URL link and is intended to be viewed by customers who purchased this book only. Thank you.

Final Words

Thank you again for purchasing this book!

I really hope this book is able to help you.

The next step is for you to **join our email newsletter** to receive updates on any upcoming new book releases or promotions. You can sign-up for free, and as a bonus, you will receive a free gift. Our *"Health & Fitness Mistakes You Don't Know You're Making"* book! This book has been written to demystify, expose the top do's and don'ts and to finally equip you with the information you need to get in the best shape of your life. Due to the overwhelming amount of mis-information and lies told by magazines and self-proclaimed "gurus", it's becoming harder and harder to get reliable information to get in shape. As opposed to having to go through dozens of biased, unreliable and untrustworthy sources to get your health & fitness information. Everything you need to help you has been broken down in this book for you to easily follow and to immediately get results to achieve your desired fitness goals in the shortest amount of time.

Once again, to join our free email newsletter and to receive a free copy of this valuable book, please visit the link and signup now:

www.hmwpublishing.com/gift

Finally, if you enjoyed this book, then I would like to ask you for a favor, would you be kind enough to leave a review for this book? It would be greatly appreciated!

Thank you and good luck in your journey!

Self-Discipline To Exercise

The Ultimate Beginner's Guide To

Develop Lifetime Exercise Discipline

- 30 Daily Champion Strategies to

Build, Develop, Control Your

Willpower & Mental Toughness

By *Freddie Masterson*

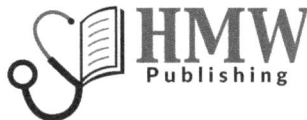

HMW Publishing

For more great books visit:

HMWPublishing.com

Table of Contents

Introduction

Every human being knows what he or she wants. Each one of us has a goal to achieve and an objective to accomplish. It is part of living. From the smallest child to the most seasoned veteran, people have in their minds something they feel can give them a real sense of meaning and identity. But along with this acknowledgment, we also need to take note of the many challenges thrown our way.

We can never control how things play up. One way or another, we will have to dwell in the uncertainties of life that would make us frown, from stepping on a wad of chewed gum to losing an apartment to a terrible fire. But in many cases, circumstances such as these are not the only things keeping you down. Mostly, you become the sole reason for your failures, and this is not something you should let live.

The fact is people who accomplish great feats owe their successes not on luck, but on the sheer ability to control their desires and to keep themselves from being complacent with what they currently have. Successes and failures should not be grounded on fortune or the lack thereof because they are more tied to how we live through self-discipline.

Most people do not realize it, but they possess a lack of self-discipline in the things they strive for. For example, people who have weight loss goals would still binge on junk food (in other words cheat) if they feel eating a small potato chip would not suddenly lead to a bloated figure. Another is how smokers keep making promises on breaking their habit, reverting after just a few days of nicotine-free lungs. Students themselves need more practice in maintaining self-discipline, particularly in studying for exams and completing projects on time.

It would be safe to say that self-discipline is a considerable factor defining our seriousness towards the goals we want to achieve. Perhaps, it could be the most significant challenge to hurdle, since the greatest enemy we have to face is ourselves.

There is a semblance of truth to that mantra. It is even true for many who seem to fail at achieving their objectives. This is because they would not dare argue with themselves over such a trivial issue.

While this book's title is "Self-Discipline To Exercise". Most, if not all, of the strategies and information that will be shared can be applied to any aspect of your life in order to stay focused and disciplined towards your goals. Keep on reading to discover how you can begin implementing theses powerful strategies to conquer any obstacles and achieve your dreams.

Also, before you get started, I recommend you **joining our email newsletter** to receive updates on any upcoming new book releases or promotions. You can sign-up for free, and as a bonus, you will receive a free gift. Our "*Health & Fitness Mistakes You Don't Know You're Making*" book! This book has been written to demystify, expose the top do's and don'ts and to finally equip you with the information you need to get in the best shape of your life. Due to the overwhelming amount of mis-information and lies told by magazines and self-proclaimed "gurus", it's becoming harder and harder to get reliable information to get in shape. As opposed to having to go through dozens of biased, unreliable and un-trustworthy sources to get your health & fitness information. Everything you need to help you has been broken down in this book for you to easily follow and to immediately get results to achieve your desired fitness goals in the shortest amount of time.

Once again, to join our free email newsletter and to receive a free copy of this valuable book, please visit the link and signup now:

www.hmwpublishing.com/gift

Chapter 1. Zap the Roadblocks Away

You begin the day by telling yourself, "I'm going to do great and important things." After you make your bed and cap you morning rituals with a hearty breakfast and a nice, hot cup of coffee, you venture off into the world with a renewed sense of wonder. It happens every day. Your journey to work with an optimistic vibe, expecting things to go your way. The printer is functioning correctly, you have a set of well-sharpened pencils, and your mind is now in serious mode, locked on the prospect of getting the promotion you deserve for working so vigorously.

The day suddenly takes a sharp curve that comes crashing into your head like an out-of-control race car. You were called by your boss who told you your performance is not good enough. You ask him how come, but he only gives a vague gesture aimed at your perceived inability to comprehend. You know you have been working so tediously for the past few months, but why peddle the idea that you are a lazy slob?

You feel you don't deserve it and you have this image of your fist planted on the boss' face. But then again, something hit you first. Looking back on the past few weeks, you realize you have been doing mediocre work all this time, and what transpired in the boss' office suddenly makes sense.

So you see, realizations such as this happens almost every day because people are inclined to expect the good from themselves. We have specific goals to accomplish, and we take it to heart to achieve them.

Then again, we encounter several obstructions along the way. And their sole purpose is to prevent us from reaching point B. Your boss probably senses the mediocre output you gave and called your attention. You are basically what he terms as a slacker, a worker epitomizing the kind of laid-back attitude subverting office culture. In a word, you are what he calls "inefficient."

And that right is a nail to the heart and the ego. So, what went wrong? You feel you did an excellent job, but your overconfidence went beyond the actual work you do.

One of the greatest roadblocks to achieving a well-balanced and disciplined life is bravado.

And there are other reasons as well, and they all seek to present promises of comfort but provide reasons to put any prospect of reaching your goals at risk.

Many people usually deny being a procrastinator or a lazy worker, but that is because they were focused more on results than implementation. That is where most individuals fail to realize. Nothing ever comes true until you set out towards doing it. But then you have several barriers along the way, so what should one do?

Let us try to dissect these barriers and provide the suitable courses of action to take in addressing these:

1. Procrastination

Let's face it. We have this knack of putting off a task. It is a disease that continues to haunt office spaces and classrooms.

Procrastination is a condition manifesting time and again to impede any step towards progress. For a fact, we can never deny looking at a problem, shrugging our shoulders, and telling ourselves we have enough time to finish it. But when the deadline nears, we find ourselves in a predicament where regret gradually engulfs us and our sanity fades into limbo. Working in the last minute is what most people prefer, saying it is a natural way of taking life less seriously until they realize the trouble they peddled using this logic.

True. However, successes do not always appear out of nowhere. They should come from somewhere, and that somewhere is our ability to spring into action. So, if you are serious about leading a life full of opportunities, you need first to understand the importance of "doing" rather than waiting.

We all know the effect of procrastination, and it is difficult to address efficiently. It comes with the fact that we always strive for the comfortable road towards life-building, yet this very notion does not play well with new rules.

Our society today is ruled by the permanence of instantaneous action. We want things to happen fast. We have technology that evolves every year. People's tastes for products from smartphones to plastic dressers change, requiring companies to pay heed to such demands for the sake of keeping themselves afloat.

And it is without question that procrastination is mediocrity's dorm mate. Both share an indifference to work and both work to expand that indifference. Since you cannot gain anything by having them around, it would only be logical to kick them out of the house for good.

And how can we go about it? It is just a simple matter of looking beyond the present. A goal is nothing but a mirage if you lay on the sand, fuelled by the hope of having this image of an oasis in front of you. You need to get up and reach for it until it vanishes in a torrent of sand and broken dreams.

2. Distractions

Another thing to watch out for is your inability to focus on the task. Much like procrastination, distractions strive to prevent you from accomplishing what needs to be done. You may have started a project with enough vigor to pull you through, but the fact remains you are vulnerable to having your attention taken away by a YouTube video. Later on, you would be scanning several more videos, wasting precious time supposedly dedicated to serious work.

Distractions do not only manifest in such facades. They also come in utterly complex forms. They take the form of a concept. For instance, you have a goal in mind directing you towards a juicy executive position you always imagined yourself in when you were a child. The thought alone puts your mind to work. You become so eager to accomplish this goal, until a particular want for something, say pursuing a more relaxed work environment, suddenly pops up and interferes your daily tasks. Because this concept pervades your mind, you gradually lose grip with your original goal, which actually requires you to work beyond your limits to achieve. You are distracted from taking a more serious looking at your dreams.

Failures develop from such a scenario, and it allows a great deal of overthinking. People begin to regret having been distracted, seeking for techniques they could have applied to minimize the distractions.

It is just a simple matter of setting a goal and holding on to it as if it were the only thing defining your life. Your goal makes you who you are, and if you allow yourself to diverge from the path leading to it, you will find yourself sitting alone at the crossroads, wondering where to go.

3. Lack of motivation

While both of the above factors drag you down, the lack of motivation is something sucking you dry of any willingness to become someone.

Everyone has something or someone that acts as a counterweight to their trebuchet. The analogy is not at all distant from explaining the fact that a trebuchet requires a larger boulder to pull a beam and throw a missile at a castle wall. Of course, the heavier the counterweight, the farther the payload travels.

It bodes true to motivation. When we have enough support of any form acting as a counterweight, we would be more confident of achieving what we ought to. Nothing stops a motivated man from getting what he wants.

But what happens when one's motivation vanishes? For that, we need only to look at a ship without sails, drifting aimlessly in the lonely sea. It is easy to say that the absence of motivation leads to idleness, and that is true, for people need an image in their heads that should put them to work with meaning.

Everyone undergoes those moments where they feel like not working because they lack an essential ingredient that should have given them the power to control their destiny. We can look no further for a practical solution than the simple matter of finding motivation.

It could be anything or anyone, as long as it allows you to push ahead, make things possible, and ultimately, train you to become more skilled and disciplined in manning your own ship.

Chapter 2. How SMART are Your Goals?

Anyone who has had experienced management at some point came across the word SMART.

But what is SMART to the ordinary Joe anyway?

Well, SMART is an acronym taken as a principle behind success. Whatever it is we are working on; it has to be SMART. It has to have the essential qualities that indicate quality work and dedication to a perceived goal.

Now, let us dissect and discover what SMART actually means.

1. Specific

Let us face the fact that we need to focus on the things that matter. Whether preparing a project for work or realizing a personal work, we need to put in our minds the thing we want to pursue. Why follow a map when there is no telling what it is you are looking for.

In many cases, people tend to act rather than make clear the very idea they want to realize. This leads them to a fruitless quest for nothing. It is very unfortunate for some to exert so much effort only to be dissatisfied in the end. Nothing really matters when for a fact they do; it is just a matter of directing your attention to the concept in your head. When making a plan, try to think about the objectives you want to achieve. Think about it first; going about it will follow.

2. Measurable

For a fact, plans should have a measurable character. What this means is that you need a type of metric to know how much you are progressing and how much you are regressing.

Not all plans end up as intended. For instance, when starting up a business, you need to understand that there are variables involved across various aspects in managing a business. You need to calculate your operating expenses against your net profits. You also need to figure out the best marketing techniques to attract customers. And you also need to track the growth of the business over the course of time. This allows you to some measure of control with how your plan or idea is catching on, enabling you to see what is wrong with it and implement the proper solutions for improving it.

Measurability is thus crucial if you want to see the success of a plan or idea through.

3. Achievable

In all aspects of realizing an important idea or concept, you need to gauge how much of an attainable endeavor it would be

For instance, an idea of a useful and marketable product hits you, and you set about drawing it from the mind and into the real world. Usually, you would employ numerous devices that can help you in achieving it. So, you filter out what works best from those that won't work at all.

However, there will be times that nothing seems to come close to a viable solution to achieving the idea. In this case, the problem does not lie with the selection of the strategies but with the idea itself. Consequently, you will be led towards modifying the idea and make it more in tune with certain limits.

And that is precisely the gist of this principle. You can learn from the age-old mantra, "Know thyself; know thy limits."

4. Realistic

Aside from knowing what would be achieved in pursuing a plan, you need to know whether or not it will ever see the light of day. More importantly, you need to know if it would indeed be an endeavor that can be sustained in the long run.

Realism is vital. Managers understand this because no plan or proposition or an idea in the history of human endeavor has ever been perfect. There will be flaws and, in the most crucial aspects, there will be real-world factors and obstacles. We need to acknowledge the fact plans are not always perfect in every way, so we need to modify and change them according to how much we can achieve. We need to ground them on realistic soil. We cannot merely flaunt an idea and tell people that it is the best idea we have had. We need first to understand that material and empirical elements play into realizing them.

5. Time-bound

Planning, in some respects, has to adhere to a timetable. Notwithstanding the importance of emphasizing quality and measurability, we also need to understand that a plan has a shelf life. They have a specific target date to be accomplished.

A project does not have any serious inclination towards completing itself when the people behind it lack a deadline which motivates them. Aside from the fact that it oversees the completion of a project, a timetable also ensures that it follows through a specific, step-by-step path towards realization. We simply could not make a rush job out of a significant endeavor such as a book or an invention. We could not even afford to procrastinate and put off important work because "inspiration comes in batches." We must understand that we need to be more organized in terms of using time as a vital element to see a project through.

***With SMART in mind, you need to develop a keen sense of finding minute details about your idea. Then, using the criteria, check whether the idea is in line with each individual rubric. Once it satisfies these indicators, then you can be sure that the idea would be closer to reality.

The path to self-discipline is never just about motivational posters and self-help books. It is more about using the current material and mental resources you have to make the concepts in your head come to life.

So, before you linger on the kind of results you want to achieve, start first by analyzing what to do and what should be done to make something that is useful and efficient. Using the SMART model, you will become wiser in making crucial decisions for rousing you to action and, in effect, making a difference.

Chapter 3. Strengthening your Endurance and Tolerance

The fact of the matter is that self-discipline is never obtained through birth. It is always taught, practiced, applied and improved. As humans, we go through a myriad of experiences as we live our lives. And at each instance, people acquire new knowledge whose value realizes itself in unique, and often peculiar situations.

Our past rules our conduct. This means that every little thing we do regardless of the consequences they entail is our past trying to resurrect itself. We are always beholden to our personal histories, tied so much to it that we can never fully sever the present from them.

And this often serves as a weakness among most people nowadays. Because past situations dictate them, it does not mean that the result of this would lead to a positive end. At times, it disables us from making real progress.

Self-discipline is a project of self-development. And we mean by development as a process that involves strengthening our capacities and weakening the very foundations of failure.

Now, when it comes to self-discipline, we need to set our mind towards improving the very way we think things through. From a broader perspective, we need to figure out what makes us stronger and more capable of addressing the very situations that put us down. Endurance is critical, but in the context of self-discipline, it is something that requires extensive practice.

Apparently, not many people are capable of enduring distractions and all other elements preventing us from realizing our goals. But what they are missing out on is the fact that they can break free from this just by thinking positively and using the following techniques for preparing the self to be more disciplined in whatever it seeks to accomplish.

1. Tame your ego

Most times, we cannot help but let our ego lose, especially when we feel like it is threatened by something as trivial as an insulting remark. As humans, we cannot help but secure our reputations. It comes with centuries of traditions and customs that ultimately led to the formation of social conventions dictating who has the power and who hasn't. We are, for the most part, on the quest to relegate ourselves to a higher status.

Sometimes, it becomes more of a hindrance to greater success. Most of us feel entitled. We always strive for the best for ourselves. We know our worth, and we know that we need to realize it. So, an opportunity that comes our way instantly becomes a big ego boost. We think about how we are better than others, and we need to prove ourselves continually. But sometimes, people tend to ignore their limits. When we are given a task, we tend to do a sloppy job at it because we think we do not deserve. While this acts as if it is an emotional triumph, it actually gives a bad impression of you. And this is where you have to start re-evaluating yourself.

Start by acknowledging your limitations and knowing what you are good at. More importantly do not concentrate too much on the task per se. Focus on how you are going to finish it rather than treat your ego as if it is more important than anything. After that, try to be more considerate when it comes to the task. Finish what you must since it also provides you an opportunity to grow not just your reputation, but also your emotional intelligence.

2. Have a daily goal

When it comes to success, gradually building up towards achieving a measure of daily accomplishments is close to improving yourself.

Every time you wake up each day, put your mind on work mode at that instant. Plan your day ahead and, most important of all, set a goal you want to achieve for the day. Whether it is the number of reports you have to make or the stage of a project you are working on, once you have something to look forward to, you can be confident of setting the day on the right track.

3. Enrich yourself

One way to build endurance is not so much about undergoing a myriad of challenges on the regular. It is also about learning how to take a break. We need time to rest because, well, we are not like robots that are bereft of any feeling of tiredness.

Recreation is your time to energize, but you have to take advantage of it in terms of enriching your mind and your spirit. Immerse yourself in a good book or, if you are not into the whole literati thing, then you might as well look for educational YouTube videos which can provide you some inspiration.

Remember: We get motivated by anything, even from the unlikeliest places. Always be inspired.

4. Learn to say "No"

One thing that is difficult to do is to say "No." Apparently, most people follow certain social conventions to some degree that they extend it towards other aspects of their lives.

Saying "No" is something we seem to shun, out of the idea that we would be branded as arrogant or rude if we do. But what most people fail to realize is that saying "No" is the hallmark of a mature mind. Of course, we say yes to things, but in particular situations where it is a viable option. But when you have an inclination to say no to an idea you feel wouldn't pass as a good one, than to disagree becomes a necessity.

Sincerity is what is indeed lacking nowadays as people refuse to speak up for fear of being isolated. But a life that is full of action and indeed a disciplined life has to have that element that resists things out of sheer concern.

So, next time you are confronted by an idea you think would not work well, try to blurt out these two letters. In fact, there is really nothing rude about it since it is your very own way of saying "This needs improvement."

Ultimately, by using these ideas would make you even more emotionally prepared to take on yourself. As with the case of many successful people, maturity comes when you learn how to train your mind to become fully confident of what it wants, fully concentrated on what is to be done, and fully aware of its own power.

Chapter 4. Harness the Power of Accountability

Apparently, everything we do is aimed at a specific objective, and to accomplish this goal, we need to understand precisely what it takes to start, maintain and end.

The gist of self-discipline is more anchored on training yourself to become more resolute and confident in your decision-making. Not only that, it seeks to improve yourself in ways that allow you to become proactive and ready for life's challenges.

Regardless of where you work and what type of work you are engaged in, you need a certain amount of discipline to make a serious effort out of it. On the other hand, you need to realize first of all that starting a task, whether it be in the short or long term, you require a great deal of seriousness on your part.

This entails knowing you have a stake at the job at hand. Creating a project and overseeing its completion is not just a matter of doing something. More crucial is the fact that you are doing it due to the pressures of accountability.

We define accountability as that element gluing us to the job. When we are given a task, by a boss or by someone else, we need to underscore the very fact that there is a particular measure of trust involved.

For instance, when the group sets about working on a project, individual members are given specific tasks that ensure the project's success. No matter how small the task can be, its greater significance becomes apparent when the project finally becomes a real thing. It is for this reason that people should focus on the task given to them to make things happen.

Does this also apply to individual projects? Of course! The fact of the matter is that building an idea from scratch to finish depends on how we see it and how our actions fit into the process of realizing the full value of one's work.

Accountability is, therefore, an essential element that needs to be acknowledged solely for its value in completing a task. We all know about the various consequences of ignoring this principle. Because of a lack of a sense of accountability, people would tend to hand in mediocre work or lack any interest in making any effort in completing a task. This, apparently, leads to the very concept of laziness, and laziness gets us nowhere in life. That has already been proven by experiences we have all encountered growing up. We know what happens when we refuse to do any work. In group activities where everyone has an equal opportunity say what he or she likes, we might have come across numerous instances where we subvert our responsibilities to the group, believing that someone else would be more capable of doing the task we would have supposedly done.

So what makes for a more responsible individual? Well, for one, we need to understand the qualities of someone who takes things seriously, especially the tasks he or she is made to do.

1. Know your role

Think about it: You are not given a specific task to complete without knowing first why it was given to you. For the most part, understanding how well you fit into a group endeavor should provide with a certain level of confidence. In the long run, you are chosen for the task because you show everyone how capable you are in doing it.

Knowing your role provides you with enough insight as to your importance. Why were you chosen in the first place? Why did they give this task to you? Should someone else do it? Apparently, these questions only point to the idea that you are well-suited for the task as much as you are trusted to complete it. Accountability, hence, starts when trust is established. Do not try to break by saying things like "I'm not fit for this" or "I don't deserve this thing."

There are reasons why you are trusted, so you better complete the task or else your credibility gets smitten.

2. Train yourself to be mature

In some instances, people tend to downplay accountability on many grounds. But apparently, there is no place for immature behavior when you are faced by something as crucial as a company project or a new, marketable product.

This is not to say that we should not see the fun in everything we do. Besides, there is always an element of fun, even in serious matters. But we need to realize that modern work culture is characterized by a feeling of community and conformity to modern rules. In this, being mature in the things we do is not only a social necessity but also as a vital factor for getting things done.

A mature mind is one that can see the best in a situation and realize its own importance. It sets about working rationally to make the best out of the task you currently have. It is in this sense that you should know when fun time starts and when stringent seriousness and dedication begins.

In your case, working on a project demands the latter. There will be more time for immature activities after you see the project through. Take it as a form of compensation.

3. Be Rational

Most people tend to act on emotions rather than hear the more reasonable side of their brain when doing a task. Especially when you are a part of a group that sets about making important strides regarding relegating an idea into reality, you should be able to put your best neurones to work.

Failed projects are mostly the product of strained egos. And we all know what happens when egos are hurt. Emotional responses become the prime voice, and every time our emotional sides act up, we can barely listen to what reason has to say.

In terms of doing real work, we need to be objective. And by that, we should not allow our emotions to conquer our ability to think clearly and reasonably. Being objective is not about being condescending. It is instead a way for one to express his own opinions for the positive completion of an idea.

When you are on to something you feel would be a great testament to your capabilities as a thinking human being, being responsible is nothing but vital. Because when you know you are accountable for something, you will have to realize that there are consequences if you do not go about it in a manner that is correct.

Invoke the rational side in you and always try to see the importance of using your intellectual prowess in terms of creating something that matters.

4. Be consistently motivated

Certain times call for you to be continuously ready for action.

People with responsibilities know this because they know how valuable they are to completing a project or any endeavor for that matter. That is why they strive to seek new ways to inspire and motivate themselves. In whatever way, they always have a knack for searching an effective outlet for them to be able to do a task in the most efficient way possible.

They always find ways to enrich themselves, which is a hallmark of a life that is centered on making successful strides towards personal betterment. In the long run, the fact that they are continuously motivated means that they are also serious about doing quality work. In the course of any human endeavor, it is imperative to put a little importance on knowing what keeps you going, since this also indicates you are serious about your responsibilities.

5. Own up

Human as we are, we can never deny the fact that we can be wrong and make mistakes at times. In many cases, we feel that one little mistake is already enough of giving you a measure of pain in the butt. This is because we are so enamored by having all these responsibilities to the point of becoming self-conscious of every little thing we do.

But errors happen all the time, and there is really no perfect path towards achieving something.

The world's greatest inventions have always been subjected to numerous challenges, from the conception of an idea to implementation. But the fact remains that these ideas become real anyway because the people behind them strive to rise above their mistakes and figure out an effective way to solve every little problem that comes their way.

Stories of perseverance have always been a subject of inspiration for many. What seemed to be an inconceivable project turned out to become a real thing whose impact resonates throughout others' lives.

So, whenever you feel you did something wrong, do not delve too much on how you made a mistake. Take time to breathe and figure out the right way to move on. Always think that it is very much possible to escape a situation that seems hopeless. As long as you have an image of the very thing you want to achieve, you will be in good hands. Just maintain focus on the things that matter. Dust yourself off, accept the fact you tumbled, and continue walking. The destination is what matters, and not the fact that you made a slight stumble.

Put in mind that accountability is what matters when you want to make a serious endeavor out of the task you have at hand. Do not rely on others. You have your own self to worry about. And with that, you have your own self to depend on when things get really sticky.

Chapter 5. Visualize the Long-Term Rewards

One thing is certain, wherever we end up in the long run, we will be able to enjoy the sweet, succulent joys of success.

People are more motivated by the very idea they would reap a considerable amount of rewards in the end. Work is after all an activity that ensures returns to the one who is serious about it. You are more fixated at a job knowing that it promises substantial benefits in return.

But sometimes, anchoring our motivation on the rewards can be counterproductive. This is because people have a false notion that whatever they do would result in the compensation they want to obtain. Never mind how much work and heart you put into an idea or a task, as long as you are doing it, you are fundamentally safe. But in almost every case, this notion proves a falsehood in this era of hustling for greater opportunities.

What matters now is how you set your mind to becoming successful and putting a lot of effort into building a life that is truly the one you wanted. What most people do not get is that they tend to focus more on the rewards, distracting themselves from the actual activities that put them on the course towards achieving them.

But do not be wrong. There is nothing inimical in thinking about harvesting the fruits of your labors. It is just that most people use this thought the wrong way, resulting in them becoming misdirected. What should be done is to use the thoughts of gaining something from work as a source of inspiration, as an important ingredient that pushes you to strive for the better.

There is really nothing wrong about visualizing the rewards you want to reap. You only need to understand how to use them as a catalyst, as a proverbial energy drink that always puts you on the go.

To do this is a matter of self-discipline of course. Read the tips below to make yourself more focused towards achieving the goals you set for yourself.

1. Take time to list the things you desire

One way to keep you motivated is to have a ready list of things you want to achieve and remember that you cannot accomplish these things without applying effort in your part. It is important to know the things you genuinely want to gain as it will teach you how to become more proactive. Hard work, after all, reaps what it can.

For this, whenever you are given a task, and you do not know how to go about starting it, list down the things that would happen once you achieve it. For instance, if you are tasked to compile an industry report in a week, think about the impression your boss would give once he sees your presentation to have followed the SMART principle.

Then, think about how this impression would turn into approval as your hard work becomes acknowledged and your boss considers giving you a promotion. Such a thought should be enough to have you work better and smarter.

Once you know what you would gain from the task, it will be more evident for you to think of ways on how to make the best out of it.

2. Weigh the rewards

It would not be right to weigh the rewards before you even starting completing the task. It would be like trying to count your eggs before they hatch. We have learned from this saying since we were a child, and you know, it all makes sense! Things do not turn out the way we want them to.

Expectations face the risk of not being met, leaving us unmotivated to continue.

However, there is still some good to be drawn from this act of weighing the rewards. For instance, knowing how much opportunities you can get if you do a certain amount of work is not actually counterproductive in any way. On the contrary, it should provide the necessary conditions that allow you to accomplish the desired amount of action relative to the type or amount of rewards you will be getting once you completed your task.

Visualizing the rewards is healthy, come to think of it. Because our minds are set on perceived benefits, we are actually reinforcing ourselves to become better at doing some work. Keep calm and try to weigh the rewards if you must, if it means giving a big boost towards completing quality work.

3. Prompt yourself every day

Every day, we get distracted by the little things. Whether it be chores or recreational activities such as playing computer games, we can be certain that there are factors out there trying to impede us from realizing the goals we set for ourselves.

With that, we need to prompt ourselves every minute, to remind ourselves of the immense work we have to do. Trivial things that get us distracted are always there to bring us down and convince us that mediocrity is okay, but actually, it is not. Mediocrity breeds a life that is not suited for success, and if you already have your priorities straight, you will need to rely on the fact that you will gain a lot from being strictly focused on a task.

There will be times for recreation, yes, but when it comes to achieving the things you think will give a lot more enjoyable things than the stuff you have, then you better start reminding yourself every day of the type of life you want.

Reminders come in many forms, but nothing beats a journal that is solely dedicated to the task you want to accomplish. By recording the progress of your task, you are continually shown proximity between where you are now and where you want to be.

Another good way to remind yourself is to stand in front of the mirror and communicate with your reflection about the very thing you want to accomplish. Though this may strike you as peculiar, it is necessary if you want to zero in on your targets. Also, talking to your reflection lets you see yourself in the third person, as a different person entirely, allowing you to give a pep talk you usually would not take into heart if you keep it to your head.

Other things would minimize distractions, but the best advice you can always receive is that you need to be focused. Think about where you want to be, and you will be certain of getting there in no time.

4. Build your dreams

Everyone has a dream. Even the poorest and the most destitute have dreams. It is all part of the human experience to aspiring to something we know would give our lives a deeper meaning, affirming the notion that we are destined for something greater than we can imagine.

Dreams are only dreams because they exist in the head. You want something, and it feels good just by thinking about it. But how about doing something to make it come true? Wouldn't that be more euphoric? The fact that what was once a concept in your head is now a thing you can sense and feel proud of?

If that is the case, then it would not hurt to have you think about starting. A dream is something you should pursue, and not something you want to keep in the dark. By doing what we must to get it, we would be well off and above all, more disciplined in making things happen.

Knowing the rewards a task entails helps us come to grips with the idea that hard work leads to a better understanding about ourselves and about the way we approach an idea or a concept.

As we all know, putting effort on the basis that there is a big, hefty sum of money or a juicy promotion awaiting us is already an excellent way to make the best out of our abilities to control our desires and strive for something even greater.

Chapter 6. Get Up from the Slips Effectively

As we have learned in the previous chapter, nothing – repeat, NOTHING – comes positively. Not to put you down or anything, but one way to look at life and how we live it is to acknowledge that not all things go well. Apparently, there are several cases in which plans and ideas get subdued by unforeseen circumstances; situations that act to put any hope of becoming successful down.

The path towards success is never paved with rose petals. It is a highway filled with danger and potentials for mishaps. It is a road in which the elements try to slow you down, break your vehicle apart and ultimately prevent you from achieving your intended goals.

The image of a reward can help, but it wouldn't be enough since you need to have an entirely different mindset when encountering a trial you think you are unable to outlast. The fact of the matter is that we need to expect the unexpected. Anything terrible that might happen will happen, and we all know better than to be unprepared for such situations.

In any case, errors and mistakes might fall upon our heads and leave us hurting with a concussion in our brains. But it does not entirely mean that the journey ends there. As we have already explained, there are still opportunities for you to rise from the dangers and the challenges; there are chances in which you can pick yourself up, dust off the specks of dust on your shoulder, and solider on like nothing happened.

Self-discipline would then also entail a desire to rise from the ashes and pick up from where you have left off. It is the hallmark of any successful person to make use of his many faculties to improve himself. As with the case of many successful leaders in business, politics, and culture, failures are a crucial ingredient for success. Rather see them as moments in which we are at our weakest, we should see them as important opportunities for improvement.

Developing our talents and transporting an idea into the real world has to involve a measure of failure. Both are subject to potentially disastrous situations that can leave any sane person to his wit's end. What should be understood is that you need to make use of these failures as educational talking points. But before that, you will need to know just how to recover from a disastrous point that might shatter your self-discipline.

1. Ignore the problem

What happens when a problem confronts us? Naturally, we use our heads to solve it in ways that are efficient and properly designed. But what if the problem becomes an uncontrollable situation where the only logical way out is to face it?

Well, for this case, anyone could just shrug their shoulders and move. As simple as that. We solve problems because we need to. And to do that, we should first realize the idea that problems have their own weakness points. These are areas where we can tap and reduce a particular problem into manageable terms. But when the issue becomes a more significant challenge that requires no panacea, the only thing left to do is to accept the consequences and move on.

For instance, you might not say anything to your boss especially when he complains about the quality of work you put in the project. You can start by blaming yourself for that, and you begin to think that the verbal beating you get from the boss is well-deserved karma expressed in the modern workplace. You won't do anything except to accept the sermon like a dog who had just ripped the curtains to shreds. After that, wait for emotions to simmer down. The worst is over. Take a deep breath, return to your cubicle, and focus on what else should be done. The sermon, after all, came as a helpful way to keep you motivated, to remind you that successes come from those who demonstrate a strong willingness to make them possible.

2. Learn from your mistakes

Whenever you encounter a bad situation, do not let it put you down. Always think about how it would help you regain a sense of duty directed not only towards yourself but towards others who see your importance.

We are made to fail because we need to grow. We need to be continuously reminded that we are capable of developing ourselves each time we fall. Think about it for a second: As children, we learn by experiencing the things that we, later on, see with refined clarity. We know all too well that touching a hot iron would cause severe burns, and know all too well that misbehaving gets us nowhere. We were punished back then, but only because we need to understand that societal realities require us to filter the good from the bad. In this case, making a mistake should not be time in which you wax sentimental, believing that people have a bias towards seeing your flaws. But it is precisely the wrong things you do that allows you learn more about the world around you.

We later adapted this thinking to later life. As adults, we know all too well that being lazy and procrastinating would get us nowhere, would put us in a situation from which escape is difficult, and would only serve to nurture an attitude that refuses to acknowledge the importance of hard work.

With this, we ought to know how to make our mistakes into points in which we can learn from. We should take cues from them as they equip us with the necessary knowledge to avoid making the same mistakes again. So, whenever you feel that failure has pinned you down, analyze where you went wrong and always make sure you use what you gathered from the experience for your own self-improvement.

3. Everything gets better

True, self-discipline is more of an issue surrounding how to start. How to maintain doing something, on the other hand, is a different issue, although self-discipline still has a significant stake in it.

In all of the human endeavors, we can never live without having to think about stuff happening the opposite way. We are idealists in our own way, but our vulnerabilities point us to the bleaker side of ambition. Failures abound, and it haunts anyone who strives to cultivate a better meaning for himself. It is important for people to, first, acknowledge their faults and, second, try to understand that they are part of this grand scheme that aims to make us masters of our own lives. For the most part, the main idea is for people to think that failures exist because not everything is perfect. But we should also recognize the fact that life gets better along the way.

Uncertain is such a prevalent condition in this universe that we would rather sacrifice it for the sake of living life that is free from challenges. But what is life without the presence of the bad? Would it be as exciting as it is? Apparently not, because what makes existing beautiful is that fact that we are doing something to make ourselves more emotionally and intellectually adamant. And nothing could ever change this fact.

So, whenever you feel beaten down by the pressures of life, think about how it would become better as time passes because life is not always there to push you around. It is also there to give you a bouquet of flowers whenever it feels like it.

Give life a chance because it eventually gets better from there.

4. Build an effective emotional base

What this means is that you need to find the very people that are the source of your inspiration. For much of your life, you have met numerous personalities growing up. You learned how having a family is important since it is the very first social circle you encounter, and incidentally the most intimate, the closest to your heart. Because whenever life gets you down, you always have a ready group of people you can run to for support.

If a task or a project seems too daunting, always think that you are no island. You are not alone since you have nurtured relationships that have meaning to you, that value you for who you are. Aside from family, your closest friends also are the very people you can depend on for emotional strength. They know you all too well. They know you, probably, more than you know yourself. In this case, if you stumble while running towards your goals, you can always vent your frustrations on the people who cared and solicit their advice. They know your worth, and they know all too well that you are someone who is capable of greater things.

5. Turn to the Spiritual

Finally, aside from the people who are close to your heart, it beats to be faithful. Religion provides you with meaning, and to most people, believing in a chosen doctrine gives them the strength to overcome a problem and rise from what seems to be a hopeless situation. Faith is, after all, an element that allows people to do what they think they cannot. For this reason, you will need to find time for some healthy meditation.

Spending some alone time while trying to recover from a stressful ordeal is essential if you want to tackle the world with a renewed sense of getting things done. Retreating from worldly affairs to spend some time with your own thoughts allows you to get that needed process of rejuvenation that way you would come back to pursuing your goal better than ever. You will be able to think clearly and become more capable of approaching every problem that comes your way.

Moreover, spend some time with other spiritual people and discuss how faith has helped you throughout the many trials and challenges that tested your belief system. Doing so will allow you to be more appreciative of the very things that give you happiness. Always think about how you are going to rise from these trials with the support of your beliefs.

Some people may scoff at the idea that spirituality does nothing to help people cope with the mistakes they made, but that is because they choose not to. For the people who do adhere to a belief system, it helps to know you are not alone and you are destined for a more significant identity which the world alone could not give.

For a fact, mistakes happen for the best reasons, one of which is that they allow us to grow as better people. While we always strive for the perfection, we can never separate ourselves from the underlying fact of life, which is imperfection.

Anything can happen abruptly, often taking us by surprise. But there is only that brief gasp. We are stunned, but not for long, because after that, we find ourselves back on the path towards making ideas, goals, objectives, and projects prosper.

In essence, experiencing slips from time to time allows us a deeper insight into ourselves. It will enable us to know our weakness and strengths, providing the right conditions that will allow us to improve the areas where we source the best from us and shut out the areas where we are being pulled down.

The fact remains that we make errors from time to time, but that does not mean taking every little mistake we have done altogether would entail a sabotaged dream. On the contrary, these failures are a testament to our strength and how disciplined we are to making things in our lives possible.

As many people would say, *"Carpe Diem."* Seize the day. Do whatever you can to make your life more meaningful and engaging.

Bonus Chapter. Get to Know some Real Life Fitspiration

Fitspiration is a method in which you source inspiration from everyday life, using sayings, passages and quotations relating to the idea that improving yourself is a crucial way to getting things done. Becoming more self-disciplined is an endeavor that, for the most part, requires a great deal of fortitude to facilitate. In many cases, people would say it is hard and difficult, especially when the very person that pulls them down is themselves.

For this reason, we all need a helping hand once in a while. There is nothing better than having people around to support your pursuit of a greater life.

Let us review some of the best Fitspiration to get you through the challenges that aim to put you down.

"Think of the consequences if you do nothing."

Apparently, this is something we can all agree on. The man of action is one who knows that rewards are right there for the taking. It is only just a matter of rising and taking that crucial first step to making it possible.

"Ambition is like an addiction. Once you're in it, your body needs it".

So, what this quote suggests is the fact that when we have ambitions to secure, we are primed to making sure they are reached. Just think about it: You can never become ambitious if you do not, do anything to make it come true. But once you are focused and primed your mind on this very idea of ambition, you would feel that your body, as well as your spirit, is obligated to do everything it must to acquire it.

"Discipline is about choosing what you want now and what you want most."

This one is a perfect summation of what discipline should be. We discussed earlier that discipline is something that is trained. It is not always an innate quality, but instead, it is something we should prepare ourselves to have. Now, when we are faced by an inclination to achieve what is best for us, we should never be bothered by distraction. Our goal is for us to accomplish no matter what. We know that our personal goals are there to guide us towards realizing what we want for ourselves. And we are certain that what we want the most is the best that we can provide for ourselves.

Final Words

Thank you again for purchasing this book!

I really hope this book is able to help you.

The next step is for you to **join our email newsletter** to receive updates on any upcoming new book releases or promotions. You can sign-up for free and as a bonus, you will also receive our "*7 Fitness Mistakes You Don't Know You're Making*" book! This bonus book breaks down many of the most common fitness mistakes and will demystify many of the complexities and science of getting into shape. Having all this fitness knowledge and science organized into an actionable step-by-step book will help you get started in the right direction in your fitness journey! To join our free email newsletter and grab your free book, please visit the link and signup:

www.hmwpublishing.com/gift

Finally, if you enjoyed this book, then I would like to ask you for a favor, would you be kind enough to leave a review for this book? It would be greatly appreciated!

Thank you and good luck in your journey!

About the Co-Author

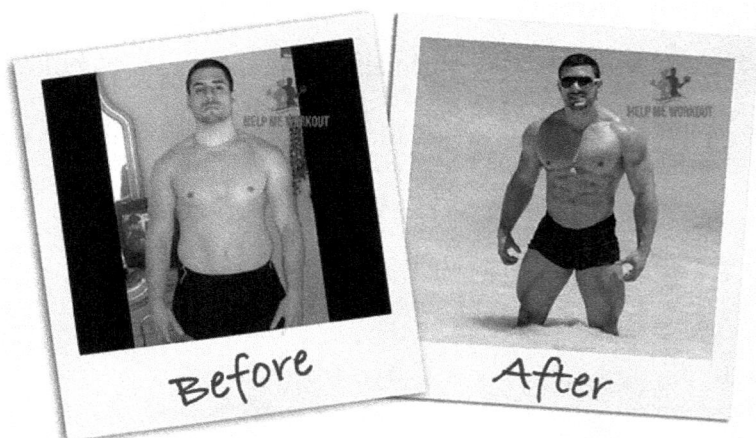

Before   After

My name is George Kaplo; I'm a certified personal trainer from Montreal, Canada. I'll start off by saying I'm not the biggest guy you will ever meet and this has never really been my goal. In fact, I started working out to overcome my biggest insecurity when I was younger, which was my self-confidence. This was due to my height measuring only 5 foot 5 inches (168cm), it pushed me down to attempt anything I ever wanted to achieve in life. You may be going through some challenges right now, or you may simply want to get fit, and I can certainly relate.

For me personally, I was always kind of interested in the

health & fitness world and wanted to gain some muscle due to the numerous bullying in my teenage years about my height and my overweight body. I figured I couldn't do anything about my height, but I sure can do something about how my body looked like. This was the beginning of my transformation journey. I had no idea where to start, but I just got started. I felt worried and afraid at times that other people would make fun of me for doing the exercises the wrong way. I always wished I had a friend that was next to me who was knowledgeable enough to help me get started and "show me the ropes."

After a lot of work, studying and countless trial and errors. Some people began to notice how I was getting more fit and how I was starting to form a keen interest in the topic. This led many friends and new faces to come to me and ask me for fitness advice. At first, it seemed odd when people asked me to help them get in shape. But what kept me going is when they started to see changes in their own body and told me it's the first time that they saw real results! From there, more people kept coming to me, and it made me realize after so much reading and studying in this field that it did help me but it also allowed me to help others. I'm now a fully certified personal trainer and have trained numerous clients to date who have achieved amazing results.

Today, my brother Alex Kaplo (also a Certified Personal Trainer) and I own & operate this publishing venture, where we bring passionate and expert authors to write about health and fitness topics. We also run an online fitness website "HelpMeWorkout.com" and I would love to connect with by inviting you to visit the website on the following page and signing up to our e-mail newsletter (you will even get a free book).

Last but not least, if you are in the position I was once in and you want some guidance, don't hesitate and ask... I'll be there to help you out!

Your friend and coach,

George Kaplo

Certified Personal Trainer

Download another book for Free

I want to thank you for purchasing this book and offer you another book (just as long and valuable as this book), "Health & Fitness Mistakes You Don't Know You're Making", completely free.

Visit the link below to signup and receive it:

www.hmwpublishing.com/gift

In this book, I will break down the most common health & fitness mistakes, you are probably committing right now, and I will reveal how you can easily get in the best shape of your life!

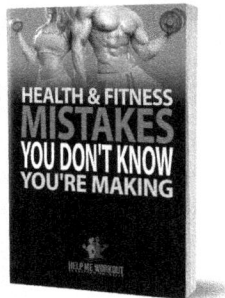

In addition to this valuable gift, you will also have an opportunity to get our new books for free, enter giveaways, and receive other valuable emails from me. Again, visit the link to sign up:

www.hmwpublishing.com/gift

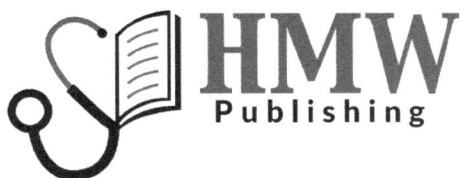

For more great books visit:

HMWPublishing.com

www.ingramcontent.com/pod-product-compliance
Lightning Source LLC
Chambersburg PA
CBHW060316030426
42336CB00011B/1079